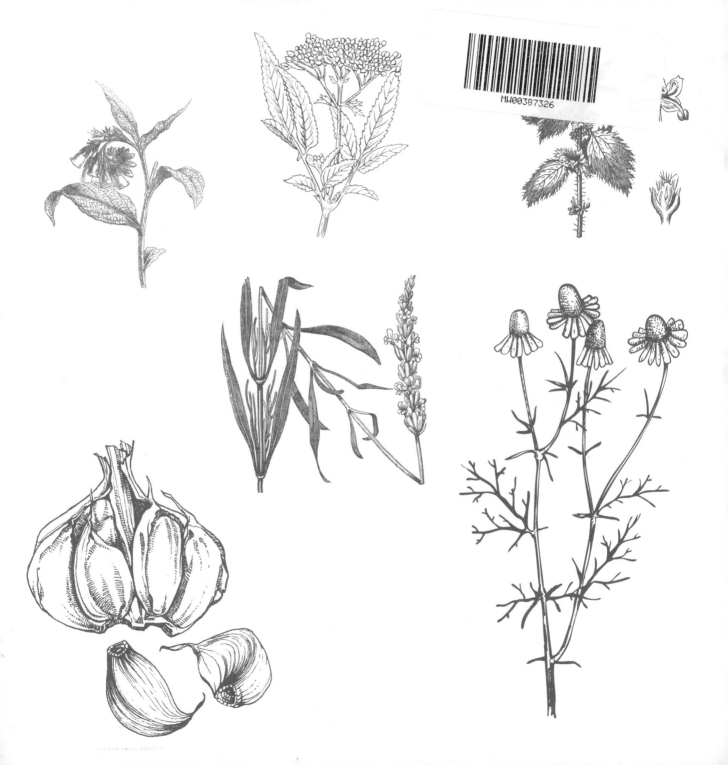

Healing Herbs

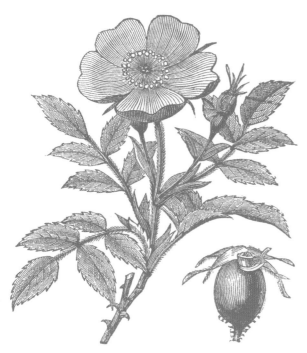

A BEGINNER'S GUIDE
TO IDENTIFYING,
FORAGING, AND USING
MEDICINAL PLANTS

Tina Sams,

editor of *The Essential Herbal*

Fair Winds Press
100 Cummings Center, Suite 406L
Beverly, MA 01915

fairwindspress.com • bodymindbeautyhealth.com

For Molly and Maryanne, my fellow woods walkers, and to all the weed workers out there who have so graciously shown me the way.

First published in the USA in 2015 by Fair Winds Press, a member of

Quarto Publishing Group USA Inc.
100 Cummings Center, Suite 406-L
Beverly, MA 01915-6101
www.fairwindspress.com

Visit **www.bodymindbeautyhealth.com**.
It's your personal guide to a happy, healthy, and extraordinary life!

18 17 16 15 14   1 2 3 4 5

ISBN: 978-1-59233-650-0

Digital edition published in 2015
eISBN: 978-1-62788-251-4

Library of Congress Cataloging-in-Publication Data
Sams, Tina.
  Healing herbs : a beginner's guide to identifying, foraging, and using medicinal
plants / Tina Sams.
     pages cm
  Includes index.
  ISBN 978-1-59233-650-0 -- ISBN 978-1-62788-251-4 (eISBN)
  1. Herbs--Therapeutic use. 2. Herbs--Identification. I. Title.

RM666.H33S256 2015
615.3'21--dc23   2014025085

Photography by Shutterstock and iStock with the exception of page 31, Susan Hess; pages 66, 113, Tina Sams
Cover and book design by Laura Shaw Design, lshawdesign.com

Printed and bound in China

The information in this book is for educational purposes only. It is not intended to replace the advice of a physician or medical practitioner. Please see your health care provider before beginning any new health program.

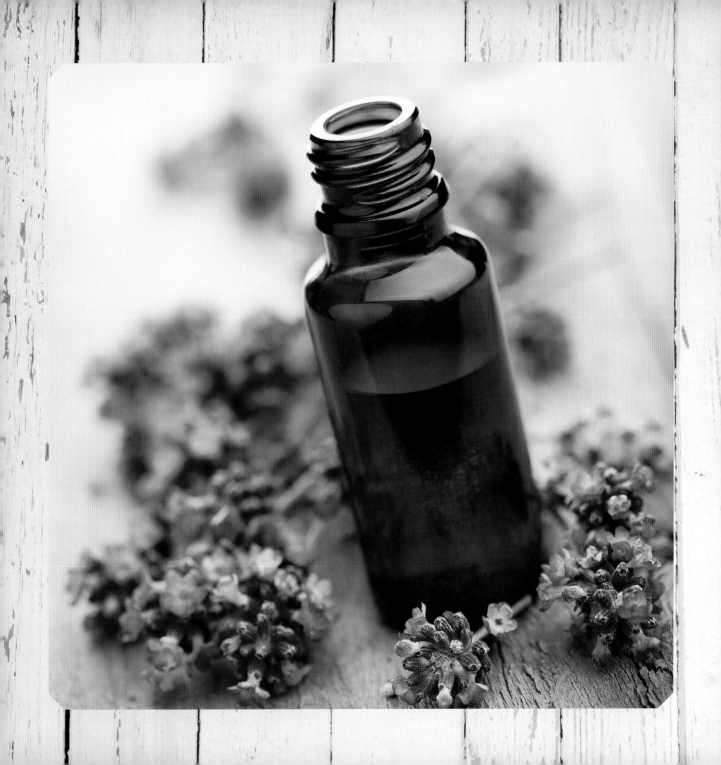

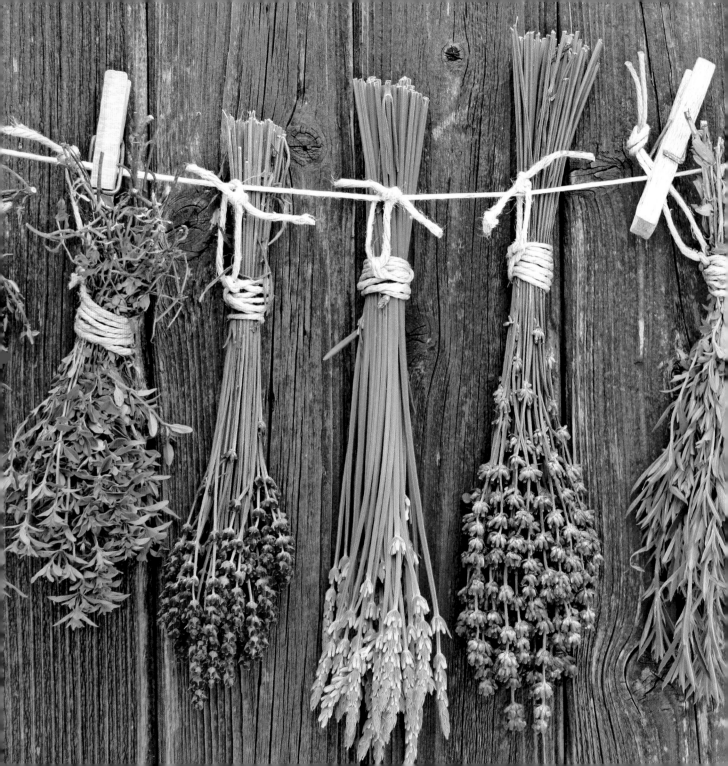

Contents

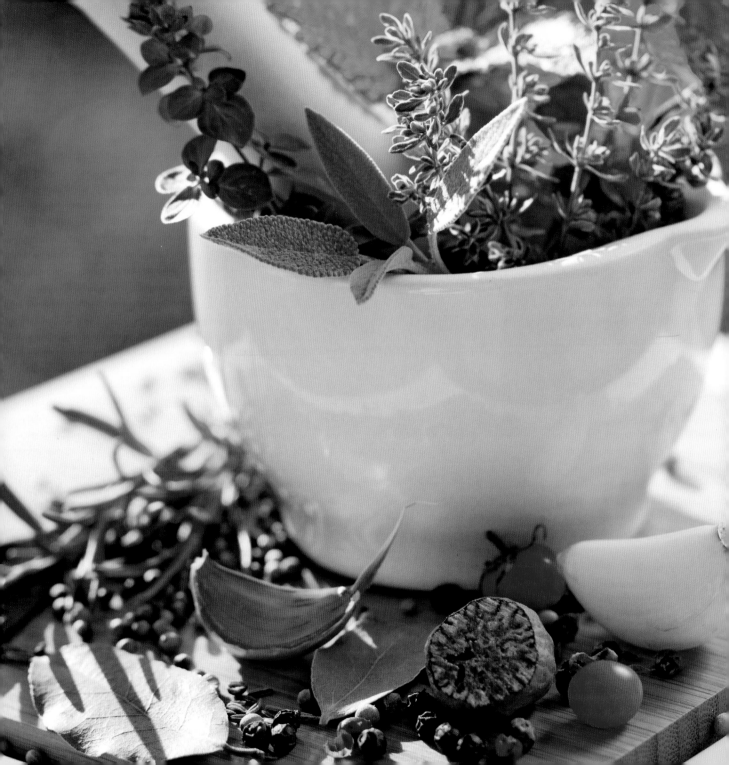

Introduction ✃

THE ROOTS OF HERBALISM extend deeper than the history of humankind. Everything that we know today follows the threads from the very beginning, woven together into a tapestry of knowledge that we tend to take for granted. Yet it is natural to seek out plants for medicine, as animals do. From the family dog eating grass for a sour stomach to chimps choosing medicinal plants for specific purposes (pain, parasites, etc.), there is a good deal of evidence that animals and humans alike turn to plants for healing. We hold innate knowledge that is often forgotten and ignored.

With the modernization of medicine, village herbalists were shunned. As an example, herbal healers in my own Pennsylvania-German region followed what is locally known as Pow-wow, or more properly, Braucherei. It is a combination of Native American healing, old German medicine, and prayer that many of the old-timers around here remember as a life-saving medicinal method, when conventional medicine failed. In the 1950s it was driven underground, as were most regional healing traditions around the world, as conventional medicine was embraced. Only in the last decade have individuals begun to work on preserving and protecting these traditions. Although some herbal healing modalities in countries such as India and China have flourished, even there the rural herbalists are currently working with people who are documenting their work and the herbs they use. In the Amazonian rainforests, researchers are racing to learn from the village herbalists before time runs out. This work is being carried out around the world as our elders pass on and we realize how very soon it can be lost forever or lost to deforestation.

As a child, I spent every possible moment outside. The plants were our toys, our companions, and our building materials. We knew what we could eat, what was poisonous, and what would cause our skin to blister. Despite the distractions of television, the Internet, and other technology, it gives me hope to see young parents encouraging their children to appreciate and enjoy the natural world. More and more parents are teaching children to find wild foods to nibble, plants to soothe a sting, and how a soft bed of pine needles on the forest floor can be the perfect place to while away an afternoon, watching the birds and the clouds.

Herbal traditions have been passed down through generations as parents and grandparents teach it to their children. That is how it has been sustained. Currently, there are many learning opportunities available without the barriers of space and time, thanks to herbalists using the Internet as a teaching tool. There is no substitute for hands-on work with the plants, however.

I started out with a good background from growing up in an agrarian region with an unquenchable desire to learn what herbs could do. My sister and I would each read a different book on herbs, switch and read the other, and then spend a week or two discussing them. I spent winters pouring over piles of field guides until the information was memorized and the pictures were as familiar as those of friends and relatives. Next came years of working with the various kinds of preparations that are made with herbs—teas, tinctures, salves, soaps, and all kinds of infusions using different menstruums (solvents). Rounding up guinea pigs was not always so easy, but gradually getting to witness the miraculous healing properties of the herbs and the things I made with them gave me more and more confidence to continue learning and using them. It wasn't long before people would come looking to me for a salve or a syrup.

After opening an herb shop with my sister in the early 1990s, the education began in earnest, as we were immersed in herbs all day, every day, and found ourselves surrounded by other herbalists with new ideas and inspirations. Herbal education is ongoing. You can never know "everything," but knowing five or ten herbs well is enough to make a difference, and will set you on the endless quest to know more.

If you are a person who loves plants, I can promise you that there will be few things in life as rewarding as learning how to use herbs in all of their aspects.

GETTING STARTED

One of the most difficult things about learning how to use herbs, whether for cooking, medicine, or a combination, is the sheer number of them. You decide to start learning about herbs and are faced with hundreds of unfamiliar plants, some with strange names that you've never heard. How will you ever learn all of those plants without confusing a poisonous lookalike? How will you learn all of those quaint terms and concoctions? Where does one even begin?

The most important thing to remember is that most herbalists use ten or fewer herbs 90 percent of the time. Getting to know one or two really well at a time can make a huge difference. It's the same with wild food foraging. Think of all the vegetables available to us. How many do you really eat, though? For most people, that's close to ten. Adding three or four wild vegetables expands the palate immensely.

Start by reading a few field guides; winter is an excellent time to review them. I expect by spring you'll have a few herbs that you'll be anxious to find and use. You'll learn what kind of terrain it can be found in, what it would look like from a distance and up close, and what kinds of plants might be found nearby.

One of the very first ones I researched was bittersweet. I wanted to use the rustic vines and vibrant red and orange berries to make a wreath. I was certain that it would be in our woods somewhere, so off I went, into the chilly early winter air to search. It just had to be in there. After about an hour, it was time to give up and rethink the plan. Turning to head home my foot slipped on the steep, wet bank of the creek, and I slid down into the shallow water. Grabbing onto exposed tree roots to climb out, I looked down at the dirt next to my hands and laughed out loud, seeing bittersweet berries scattered all around me. Leaning back to look up, I saw that the vines were high up in the trees, much further up than I'd looked before. The research had not let me down.

The following year, chamomile caught my eye. The year after that it was elderberry. And so it went. Springtime will find me a true menace on the roadways; I've been known to frighten companions with screams of recognition and leap from a not-entirely-stopped vehicle at the sight of a field of trillium.

I recommend finding one or two new plants each year. Find them, sit with them, and observe them throughout the growing season. Use them. Make them into every kind of preparation you can think of that makes sense. Cook with them, make them into salve, a tincture, a tea, a bath blend, or a syrup. Try using the different useful parts of the plant and comparing the qualities you find. In other words, get to know them thoroughly so that you could find them in the dark by their scent, growing habit, and neighbors. Once you know them, they will be a part of your herbal repertoire forever.

RESPONSIBLE WILDCRAFTING

There are a few things to think about when gathering plants from the wild.

» Be absolutely certain in your plant identification.

» Take no more than you need, and never harvest if there is not an abundant supply of the plant. Even in abundance, take no more than one-quarter of the stand, cutting in such a way that the plant will regrow if possible. Roots should be taken with the utmost care, and if there are seeds that are not your objective, return them to the ground. In my yard, dandelion, violets, and chickweed, when harvested, are so prevalent that this is not necessary, but until you know what needs conservation, exercise restraint.

» Do learn about the endangered plants list and leave the struggling ones alone. You can find this information at United Plant Savers, www.unitedplantsavers.org.

» Stay at least 100 feet (30 m) back from roads and railroad tracks. If you've ever watched a snowplow throw snow, you know it really travels. There are also issues of exhaust, runoff, and chemical spraying to reduce weeds by local jurisdictions. The farther away, the better.

» Getting permission from the landowner is the right thing to do. Considering that what you want will usually be a weed, it is rare to be turned down. Even in the case of old fruit trees or medicinal trees, most landowners will be generous. It also gives you a chance to find out whether they have been treated with any chemicals that you don't want.

» Let someone else do the driving so you can focus on identifying plants you pass. Enjoy watching the verdant awakening outside the window, and plot your next wildcrafting adventure.

BASICS OF MAKING HOME REMEDIES

Salve/Balm/Ointment

A salve (also often called a balm) is an oil or a fat combined with a small quantity of wax (usually beeswax) to obtain a specific consistency. The amount of wax used is what determines the hardness or looseness of the salve. If a loose salve is desired, very little wax is used. If the salve is being made to hold a shape like lip balm or a lotion bar, more wax is used.

The first salve I ever made was intended as a prank gift for a male friend mourning his upcoming fortieth birthday. My sister and I slowly simmered specific herbs in hydrogenated soybean oil, strained it, and did not add any wax at all. We name it "Forever Young" salve, and instead of chuckling at our little ribbing, he was delighted and used it.

Below is a general list of ratios for creating salves and balms:

	Base Oil	Wax
Salve/Ointment	6–8	1
Lip Balm	3	1
Lotion Bar	2	1

Infusing Oil for Salve, Balm, or Lotion

Often, the oil or fat used in the preparation has been infused with an herb or a blend of herbs for a specific purpose. There are a lot of ways to do this, but I'm not the patient type. If the herbs are fresh, allow them to wilt and release some of the water they hold.

You can also use dried herbs. If you have an oven with a warm setting, that's a great place to infuse the oils, and I like using a slow cooker, too. Some feel that the slow cooker is too hot and so they install a rheostat; others all but deep fry their herbs. Some use sunlight over a period of several weeks (no lid, covered with a secured cloth) but occasions of mold growing have turned me away from that method. I like "low and slow" myself.

Keep in mind that the herbs will absorb some of the oil, so when you strain them be prepared to squeeze them out well. I personally hang on to worn-out T-shirts and cut them into 8-inch (20.3 cm) squares. They fit into the colander and strain things much more quickly than paper coffee filters. Then I pick up the cloth square by the corners and squeeze all the good herb-rich oil out.

Tip: When melting wax, combine it with about one-fourth of the oil (for small batches, less for larger batches) until melted and then add the rest of the oil to combine. Otherwise, the wax will harden immediately when the cooler oil hits it. This way, you don't need to heat all of the oil hot enough to melt the wax.

Tip: Work in small quantities. Rarely will you need more than 4 ounces (115 g) of anything unless you're making gifts. The first trial batch of anything can be less than 1 ounce (28 g) and is plenty to try.

Syrup

There are a couple of ways to make syrup. Both begin with a strong herbal infusion or tea. Brew the herb(s) in just boiled water for at least 15 minutes and up to an hour. Strain.

METHOD #1

1 cup (235 ml) strong herbal tea

2 cups (400 g) sugar

¼ cup (60 ml) vodka or brandy (optional)

Heat the tea while stirring the sugar to dissolve. When it reaches a boil, allow it to boil hard for 3 minutes. Skim off any scum. Add the vodka to help it remain shelf-stable longer. Pour into a sterilized bottle and store in the refrigerator until needed. The syrup should keep up to 6 months.

Yield: 2¼ cups (530 ml)

METHOD #2

1 cup (235 ml) strong herbal tea
1 cup (320 g) honey
¼ cup (60 ml) vodka or brandy (optional)

Heat the tea and honey gently to combine. Add the vodka to help it remain shelf-stable longer. Pour into a sterilized bottle and store in the refrigerator until needed.

Yield: 2¼ cups (530 ml)

Tincture

It is best to make tinctures individually. A tincture made with a single herb is called a "simple," and it can then be blended with other tinctures in smaller quantities for a more specific remedy if need be. There is nothing wrong with blending herbs to make a tincture, but you are then stuck with that blend when you might just want the single herb for something. Some plants, especially roots, will leave a white, milky residue. It is inulin, a naturally occurring carbohydrate present in more than 36,000 plants; it is not a problem.

I have never seen a tincture "go off." The alcohol is a strong preservative. Even though you may see expiration dates on commercially sold tinctures, they are only there because producers are required to come up with one. One producer told me that he chose ten years, arbitrarily. The alcohol used is entirely up to you.

I find that 80 to 100 proof is best as a solvent to pull the medicinal components from the plant material. Grain alcohol (190 proof) is good for some things, but most plants have water-soluble components as well as alcohol-soluble components, so it is often too strong. I have friends who like to use whiskey, and one who swears by Southern Comfort for all her tinctures. Lots of people use brandy. I don't mind admitting that I've been caught on occasion with a plant that needs tincturing and only something like rum or gin in the house. It works.

The folk method of making a tincture is almost too simple to believe.

USING FRESH HERBS:
1 pint (470 ml) canning jar
Enough fresh (best to allow to wilt for a few hours) plant material to loosely fill jar
Alcohol to cover (I generally use 100 proof vodka)

USING DRIED HERBS:
1 pint (470 ml) canning jar
Enough plant material to fill the jar one-fourth to one-third
Alcohol to cover (I generally use 100 proof vodka)

Add all the ingredients to the jar, put the lid on the jar, and allow it to steep 4 to 6 weeks, shaking it once a day.

After it is finished, you may strain it or leave as is until needed. A pint jar will yield anywhere from 1 to 2 cups (235 to 470 ml), depending on the herb used and how absorbent it is, but most families find that a pint of just about anything is plenty for a year or two.

For most herbs, a dropperful is approximately equivalent to a strong cup of herbal tea.

Yield: 1 to 2 cups (235 to 470 ml)

Herbal Tea

Teas (also referred to as infusions) are an excellent, enjoyable way to use herbs. Many people are intimidated about blending teas but need not be.

I often tell the story of my first year of wildcrafting. Everywhere I went, I carried little bags and if I saw something that I'd read could be used in tea, I gathered a handful to be dried and added to a gallon jar. I had wild rose petals, raspberry leaves, chickweed, thyme, cornflower petals, beebalm, pineapple sage, five or six kinds of mint, echinacea, elder flowers and berries, marshmallow, calendula, sage, nettles, oat straw, lemon verbena, basil, violet flowers and leaves, lavender, and probably another twenty-five ingredients by the end of summer, collected in the jar. I added a small handful of stevia, some licorice bits, some cinnamon pieces, and dried citrus peels. All winter long, we drank from that jar. Every single cup was different, usually with completely unique ingredients, but no cup was less than wonderful. It was a great lesson for me and relieved me of the stress that so many of my herbal friends go through trying to put a tea together.

A few important notes about herbal teas:

» A single herb steeped in water by itself is called a tisane.

» The leaves and flowers of an herb are steeped for about 5 minutes to make tea.

» Roots and berries are decocted, which means they need to be simmered for 15 minutes to release their flavor and medicine.

» For fresh herbs, use 1 tablespoon (4 g) per cup (235 ml) of hot water.

» For dried herbs, use 1 teaspoon (1.3 g) per cup (235 ml) of hot water.

» A nourishing infusion is made from specific herbs (stinging nettle, red clover, and oat straw in particular) that contain lots of minerals and vitamins. Add 1 ounce (28 g) of the dried herb to a quart (1 L) jar, pour boiling water over it, place the lid across the mouth of the jar to retain the heat/steam, and let it steep overnight. Drink the resulting concentrated infusion during the course of the day.

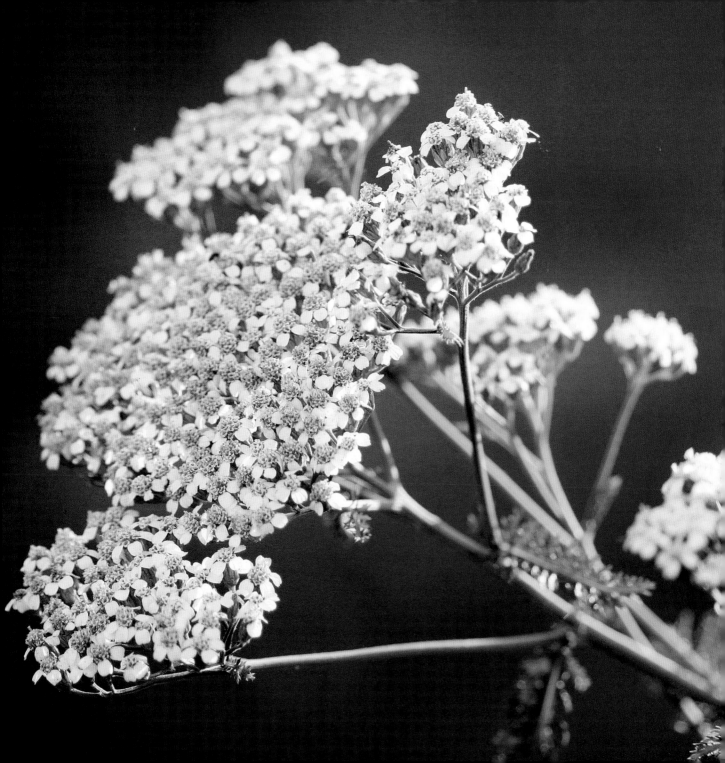

CHAPTER ONE

Yarrow

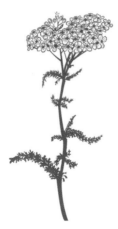

Achillea millefolium

Asteraceae family

SOFT FERNY LEAVES and delicate yet firm, compact flower clusters form on the erect stems. These perennials are mostly white flowered in the wild, with some tinged pink. The bright yellow, salmon, and red available at garden centers also have medicinal properties, but are bred for color. As is typically the case, the wild or common variety is the one we choose for medicine. That which is closest to nature has the most perfect content to heal. Although there are exceptions to every rule, it seems that once humans start trying to extract specific properties, we throw off the balance of things.

Daniel Gagnon of Herbs, Etc. once gave a seminar about standardized herbal remedies, and I was very drawn to his metaphor of plants being like symphonies. We need all of the instruments to enhance, buffer, and activate each other to fully enjoy the music. So it is with plants. While it may be more convenient to breed away the thorns or prettier to view the deep scarlet blossom rather than the white, when hunting for medicine or food, it's usually best to use the original. In fact, I suspect this topic will become quite important over the next twenty years with regard to our food plants.

Yarrow is one of those plants that did not initially call to me. I do think it is beautiful, and its long and mythical history is beautiful, but it just kept growing closer and closer to my house. Different herbalist friends spoke of their fondness for yarrow, some proclaiming it to be their very favorite (a distinction that is very rare for any herb), and still I looked on while it marched across my yard. It now makes up nearly half of my front yard, although it is neatly mowed most of the time. Instead of grass, I have a short, lacy mat of yarrow leaves. In spite of never getting a chance to bloom, it seems happy. Perhaps it was time to start paying attention. As has often been the case, when the herb comes calling, I listen and begin to learn about what it has to offer.

Yarrow is an ancient herb, said to get its name, *Achillea millefolium*, from Achilles. Legend has it that Achilles had become a great healer under the tutelage of the centaur Cheron, and yarrow was one of his great herbal allies that he used to staunch the bleeding wounds of his fellow soldiers in battle. Nicknames like soldier's woundwort, knight's milfoil (not to mention many others—nosebleed, devil's nettle, and old man's pepper among them) come from this. The species name, millefolium, and one of the common nicknames for yarrow—milfoil—means "thousand leaves" and comes from the fact that the feathery leaves of yarrow actually appear to be made up of many tiny leaves.

In China, yarrow is also used for divination. The ancient oracle of the *I Ching* is traditionally

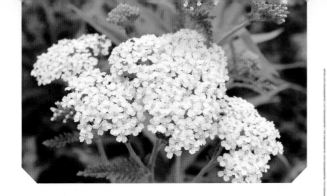

cast with yarrow stalks, thought to represent the yin and yang forces of the universe in perfect balance.

Yarrow is best known as a styptic or vulnerary herb, useful in stopping bleeding. The juice or dried herb powder can be applied to bleeding wounds, or in the field fresh plant material is used. Not only is this used externally, but also strong infusions may be drunk for internal bleeding. Depending on the issue, other herbs can be blended with yarrow to soothe the tissues. Yarrow is anti-inflammatory, too; it contains salicylic acid derivatives, making it useful for fever and reducing pain. Relaxing to the voluntary nervous system, yarrow tea can help with all manner of cramping and spasms, particularly uterine (so check with your physician if pregnant). Stomach cramps are also responsive to yarrow, and since it is a bitter herb, it helps with digestion and is a tonic to the liver and gallbladder. It can stimulate a flagging appetite, and help with indigestion and heartburn. Traditionally, yarrow has been used for insomnia and to relieve stress or anxiety. It's perfect as a woman's herb, as it is a diuretic that normalizes menses, relieves painful periods and cramps, and reduces excessive bleeding. Who needs an over-the-counter medication when yarrow is waiting right outside? Many of those same properties make it a good friend to the urinary system, relieving inflammation and pain and increasing urinary output. A blend with goldenrod would be a great choice for bladder infections and even kidney stones. Yarrow tea has long been a remedy for colds. The hot tea is diaphoretic, bringing on a sweat that breaks the fever while flushing toxins from the system. Yarrow is astringent and can be used for diarrhea as well as to shrink swollen hemorrhoids.

Medicinal Benefits

» Stops bleeding
» Reduces inflammation
» Reduces fever
» Relieves pain
» Relieves cramping
» Eases anxiety
» Astringent

COLD EASE TEA

You might notice that I like to add ginger to a lot of remedies, and this traditional tea to fight colds is no exception. The ginger and elderberries make it more flavorful and effective in my experience. I'm not keen on dried ginger pieces and fresh ginger can't go into dried mixes, so the crystallized pieces work very well. This combination will likely bring on a sweat and the peppermint will help clear the head. If you happen to have some honeyed lemons (see note), add a spoonful to the cup just prior to serving.

Ingredients

1 tablespoon yarrow
1 tablespoon elderflowers
1 tablespoon peppermint
2 teaspoons elderberries
2 teaspoons minced crystallized ginger

Directions

Combine the herbs and steep a heaping teaspoonful in a cup of water for at least 5 minutes before drinking.

Yield » Enough for 9 or 10 cups (2115 or 2350 ml) of tea

Note

Honeyed Lemons: Use organic lemons if at all possible; I prefer Meyer lemons when I can find them. My little tree only gives me a couple per year so far. Slice the lemons as thinly as possible, removing seeds as you go. Fill a jar with the lemon slices. Cover completely with honey, and refrigerate. In a few weeks, this will turn into a sweet lemon honey with portions that are almost a jellylike consistency. I can barely resist it long enough to save it for my teas!

TUB TEA FOR HEMORRHOIDS AND ITCHY BUTT

This is no laughing matter if it is bothering you. Sometimes a nice warm bath is just the thing to set things right, although it will be more of a temporary fix. Soothing the burning and itch of hemorrhoids can mean a good night's sleep, and this just may set you on the road to feeling better, along with some dietary changes. Tarragon is added to this because it has a slight numbing effect. If you nibble on a fresh tarragon leaf, you'll feel the numbing sensation on your tongue. Using equal parts is fine, but the ratio isn't critical. I can easily run out back and harvest these in a few minutes' time, but if you're using dried from a purveyor of herbs, use at least 1 cup of each of these that you have available.

Ingredients

Yarrow branches
Tarragon stems
Violet leaves
Comfrey leaves

Directions

Fill a large stockpot, the bigger the better, with water almost to the top, add the herbs, and turn on the heat. When the water boils, turn the heat off and allow the herbs to steep for an hour. Strain through a colander, reserving the liquid.

Remove enough liquid to fill an ice cube tray, and freeze that for later. The ice cubes can be wrapped in a paper towel and used individually. Pour the rest of the water into the tub and fill it so that it is comfortable to sit in it for 15 minutes to half an hour with room to add hot water as necessary.

Yield » 1 bath and 12 ice cubes

BLOSSOMS AND OATMEAL FACIAL

This is a scaled-down version of a product that my sister's soap and body care company makes. Nourishing to the skin and a pleasure to use, it can be personalized with your own choice of wetting agent. Plain water is fine, but a nice hydrosol, yogurt, an egg, milk, or an oil are just a few ideas for making this your own.

Ingredients

1 tablespoon rose petals
1 tablespoon yarrow leaves and flowers
1 tablespoon calendula
2 tablespoons oatmeal
Almond meal, cosmetic clay powder, milk powder, or other botanicals (optional)

Directions

Rose petals will often resist breaking down, so begin by putting them into a food processor, or if you're like me you have a coffee grinder (or two) just for herbs and resins. Pulse to break down. Add the remaining ingredients and process until they are a fairly uniform consistency about the size of grains of sand. Transfer the mixture to an airtight container.

To use, put about a tablespoon of the mixture in a small dish, and add enough of your wetting agent to form a spreadable paste. Wash your face using your normal cleansing method, and then spread on the facial, rubbing it around to exfoliate a little bit. Leave it on for 5 minutes before rinsing and patting dry.

Yield » 4 or 5 applications

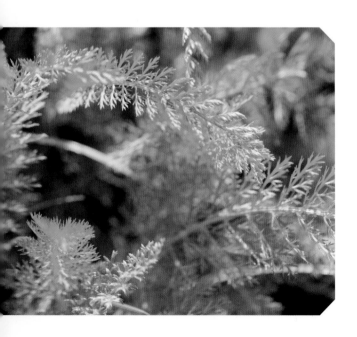

YARROW TEA

This tea is nice in winter to help poor circulation and getting warmth to cold extremities. Yarrow isn't an everyday tea to drink, though having some a few days in a row is fine.

Ingredients

⅓ **cup chopped dried yarrow**
1 quart (1 L) boiling water

Note Cautions for using yarrow:

» Yarrow intensifies the medicinal action of other herbs taken with it.

» Constant use may cause swelling of the liver.

Directions

Steep the yarrow in boiling water for about 10 minutes; this brings out just enough bitter properties to help the liver. To reduce its bitterness, use the water just before it gets to a boil. Although herbal teas are usually steeped much longer, a long-brewed yarrow tea is too bitter for nonemergencies. Store the strained herb in the fridge and brew it a few more times, quickly rinsing with very hot water first before reuse.

Drink 1 to 2 quarts (1 to 2 L) of strongly brewed tea at the onset of the flu and also drink it after encountering a person with the flu. To make a strong brew, steep 1 to 2 hours; this will be quite bitter.

Another way you can use the tea is to spray yourself with it to repel mosquitoes. Keep the tea in a spray bottle in the fridge and spray yourself all over before going out.

Source Jamie Jackson, www.MissouriHerbs.com

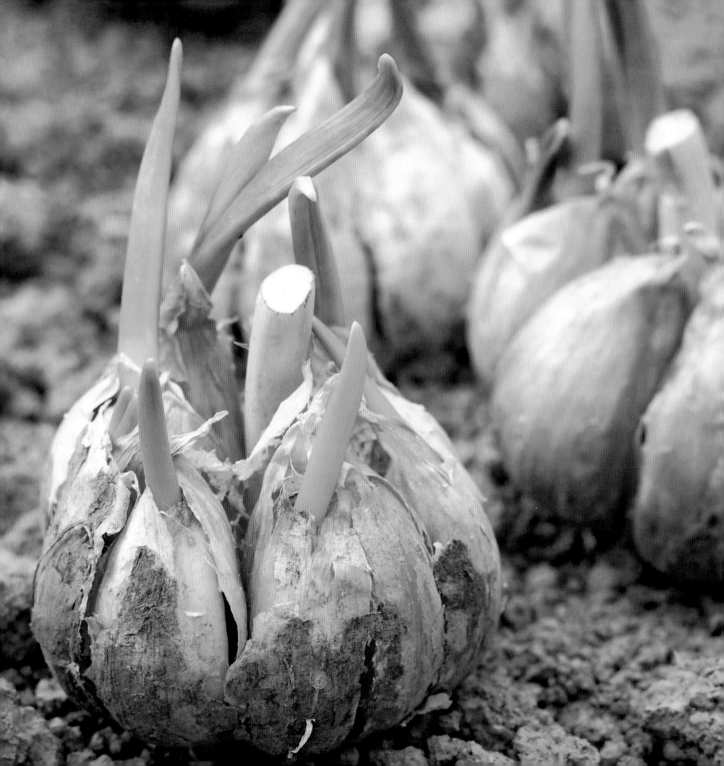

CHAPTER TWO

Garlic

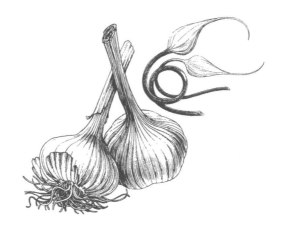

Allium sativum

Amaryllidaceae family

To many, garlic has been a typical ingredient, as common as salt and pepper on the kitchen table. Though my family rarely cooked with garlic, I would wrangle an invite to dinner with the Italian family down the road every chance I got. There was nothing that came out of my neighbors' kitchen that didn't make my mouth water upon the slightest whiff of garlicky goodness.

Garlic is a bulb composed of between four and fifteen cloves in a husk that ranges in hue from clear white to tan or even pink. Growing garlic is ridiculously easy. Find an organic source, buy a bulb, and place the cloves in the ground about 2-inches (5 cm) deep in full sun. Stalks, called "scapes," come up in early summer and are trimmed off before blooming so that the bulbs get the growth energy instead of the flower. The scapes can be used in the same way as garlic, and have recently become a sought-after vegetable.

When the cut stalks turn brown, it is time to harvest. Store in a cool, dry spot in the same way you would store onions. Many people braid the stalks and hang the garlic bulbs, removing them from the bottom as they are needed.

Garlic has been popular in folk medicine for many generations and has been in use in China, Europe, and India for eons. Even the ancient Egyptians used it for both food and medicine. It has a long, rich history, and it is no exaggeration to say that garlic is a bit of a miracle. Entire books have been written as odes to the "stinking rose," and still we continue to find more benefits from its use.

One of the best-known healing components in garlic is called allicin. The pharmaceutical crowd would move to isolate this one component and leave the rest behind, but in herbalism we know that the whole plant contains buffers and synergistic substances that activate and smooth out the effectiveness. Allicin comes in this great-tasting package, a naturally occurring antibiotic and healing powerhouse combined with enough vitamin C to prevent scurvy. There are more than 100 valuable healing components included in garlic, many of which are currently being researched.

Garlic is often used in an ear oil to help with the painful ear infections of early childhood. It has immense healing and preventive properties to fight influenza, colds, and yeasts and fungi like thrush and athlete's foot. It fights staph infection, and during World Wars I and II army medics used garlic juice–soaked moss to prevent gangrene and help fight wound infection. Crushed garlic or garlic oil can pull infection from a cut, but don't lay this simple poultice directly on the skin, as it is potent and may raise blisters. Garlic keeps us hale and hearty during our middle years with antiseptic, antibiotic, antiviral, antibacterial, and anti-inflammatory

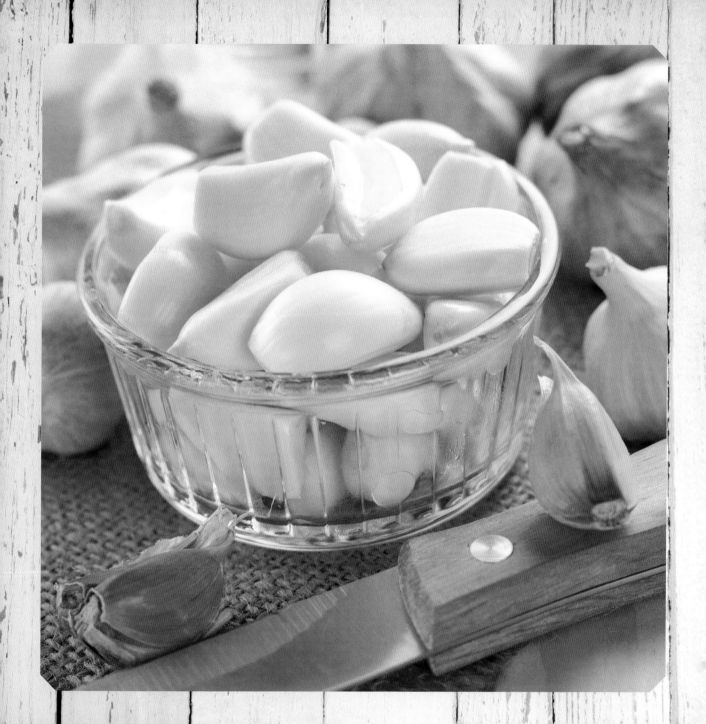

properties, and is even a repellent for worms and other parasites (however, it is toxic to household pets).

Garlic is especially useful for the elderly because it strengthens the heart and circulatory systems. It has been found to assist with high blood pressure while reducing serum cholesterol and triglyceride levels. It helps keep the blood vessels supple and free of plague. The use of garlic is very helpful in regulating levels of blood sugar, and it is potent enough that if you are using insulin and use a lot of garlic, you should let your doctor know.

It is no wonder that garlic is thought of as having the ability to ward off vampires and myriad other evils, because it actually does protect us from so many things. It is the main ingredient (along with several other potent herbs) in Four Thieves Vinegar, a renowned formula whose origin is often disputed. One story is of thieves who were able to ransack the homes of plague victims without becoming sick themselves, and when they were caught, were promised freedom in exchange for their secret; another tells of convicted thieves burying plague victims without contracting the illness themselves. A third story involves a man named Fortaves who popularized the blend, and when his name was pronounced aloud, it could easily have morphed into "four thieves." While not quite as colorful, it is probably closer to the truth. In any case, anything with so much mystery and fascination must have something going for it!

When facing viral threats, garlic is more battle-ready when consumed raw. While many people have no problem eating raw garlic, I have been researching other methods for those who prefer a less pungent remedy. With the help of a lot of garlic, I was recently able to recover from an upper respiratory infection within three days instead of the two-plus weeks that seems typical. My go-to remedy was garlic honey.

Medicinal Benefits

- » Prevents cold, flu, and fungal infections
- » Reduces skin infection
- » Kills viruses, bacteria, and other pathogens
- » Reduces inflammation
- » Lowers high blood pressure
- » Reduces high blood sugar

GARLIC HONEY

This is a fantastic remedy that I make in late summer or early fall when the local garlic and honey are both abundant. The honey is wonderful in herbal tea blends, and I fish out the garlic cloves by the spoonful to eat.

Ingredients

4 or 5 bulbs garlic
1 pint (470 ml) jar
1 pint (640 g) honey, local preferred

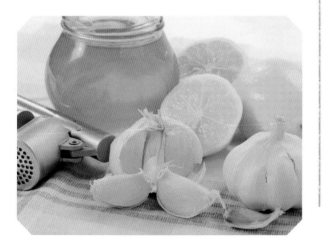

Directions

Separate the cloves of garlic, and trim the wide rough end where it attaches to the bulb. When all the cloves are trimmed, lay them out on a cutting board and holding a wide knife over them sideways, smack down with the butt of your hand or a fist. This mashes them a bit and they are released from their papery skins. Pop them out of the skins and place them in the jar.

Cover them completely with honey. They will rise to the top of the honey, and that's fine. Eventually, they'll soak up the honey and sink. Put the lidded jar in the refrigerator for at least a month. It will be there when you need it.

At the first sign of a virus, add a spoonful to a cup of tea, and repeat daily at least once for a few days until the threat is gone.

I always think that 1 pint (640 g) at the beginning of flu season will be plenty, but then I usually make a second batch in February or March because it never is.

Yield » 1 pint (640 g)

PESTO

This simple herb paste is a delicious way to enjoy some raw garlic.

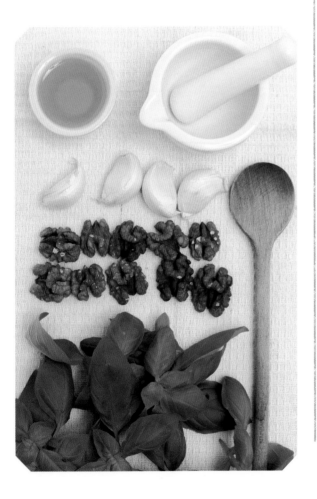

Ingredients

1 cup (60 g) basil leaves
5 or 6 cloves garlic
1 cup (100 g) grated Parmesan cheese
½ cup (75 g) walnuts
¼ cup (60 ml) olive oil

Directions

Put all of the ingredients into a food processor. Process until smooth or with a little texture; either way, it's delicious served over pasta with a few shrimp or some grilled chicken.

Yield » 1 cup (240 g)

OLIVATTA

This is a variation from one of the Moosewood *cookbooks, and is another tasty way to consume raw garlic. It is elegant enough to serve to guests, and such a nice way to help people gather and socialize during the winter and still avoid getting sick.*

Ingredients

2 cups (250 g) pitted black olives (fresh or canned)

½ bulb garlic

8 ounces (226 g) Neufchâtel or cream cheese

Directions

Place the olives and garlic in a food processor and process until coarsely chopped.

Cut the cheese into cubes, add to the food processor, and blend. Serve with crackers.

This will keep well in the refrigerator for a week or more, but you can easily halve the recipe if you're not expecting company.

Yield » 3 cups (720 g)

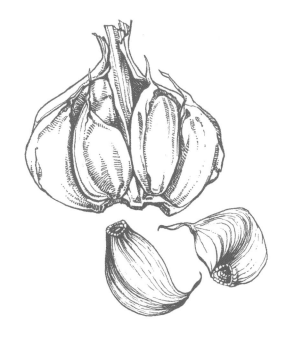

MULLEIN AND GARLIC EAR OIL

This remedy was traditionally made with sweet almond oil, and old-timers called it simply "sweet oil." This oil is not actually sweet, and I prefer to use olive oil because sweet almond has a propensity to turn rancid pretty quickly. Olive oil is also more readily available, and usually less expensive. This oil is traditionally used, slightly warmed, in children's ears during ear infections. It can also be rubbed into the soles of the feet during a cold, and then covered with thick wool socks before going to bed.

Ingredients

¼ cup (60 ml) olive oil
2 cloves garlic, minced
1 tablespoon dried and chopped mullein leaves

Directions

Combine the ingredients in a saucepan over low heat and heat gently until the oil is well warmed. You don't want it to sizzle or fry the herbs, but it should get pretty hot.

Remove from the heat and allow to steep for about 1 hour. Carefully strain the oil to remove all remnants of the herbs. A coffee filter is appropriate. Pour into a dropper bottle. Store in the refrigerator between uses to extend the shelf life. Make fresh each year.

Yield » Scant ¼ cup (60 ml)

GARLIC OXYMEL

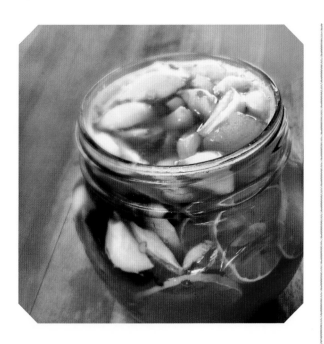

Directions

Peel and halve the garlic, thinly slice the lemon, and coarsely crush the pepper. Place in a clean glass jar. Cover with the vinegar and honey and shake until well blended.

Allow to sit for a minimum of 6 weeks. Spoon out 1 tablespoon (15 ml) at a time for a sore throat or at the onset of an upper respiratory infection. Use as needed.

This can also be mixed with a little oil and used as a delicious salad dressing.

Yield » 3 cups (835 ml)

Source

Susan Hess, www.farmatcoventry.com

Ingredients

3 bulbs garlic
1 Meyer lemon (optional)
Whole cayenne peppers, to taste (optional)
1½ cups (355 ml) raw apple cider vinegar
1½ cups (480 g) raw honey

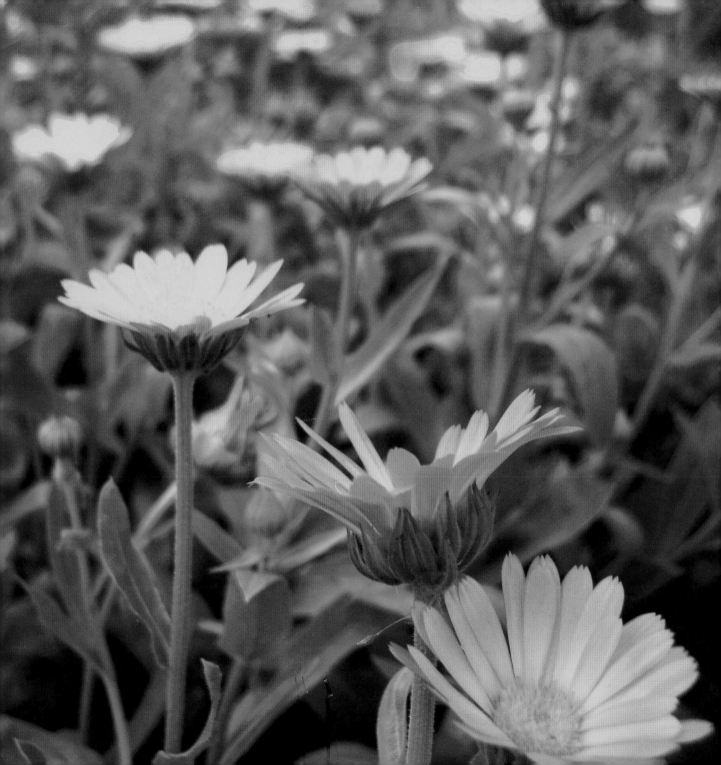

CHAPTER THREE

Calendula

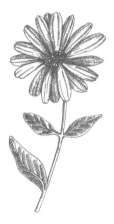

Calendula officinalis

Asteraceae family

LAST SUMMER I planted a long row of calendula in a new production garden on a hillside field. Before long, the brilliant yellow and bright orange flowers beckoned to me from the windows of the house 100 yards (91 m) away. Picking them, my hands became so sticky with the resin from the bracts, which form the green base of the flower head, that I had to stop every few minutes and scrape the petals from my fingers. The stickier they are, the more healing their medicine. The bees worked the flowers too, and I left enough for them each time. The more they are harvested, the better they produce. In fact, neglecting to keep after the flowers will allow them to set seed and the plant will shut down flower production. You cannot overpick them.

Calendula is commonly referred to as "pot marigold," a habit I would like to see go away. While calendula is a gentle, nourishing plant full of powerful healing and anti-inflammatory properties and a member of the aster (Asteraceae) family, marigolds are properly named *Tagetes* spp. and have entirely different properties. In ancient Rome it was noted that the flowers always bloomed on the first day of the month. As a result, they gave it the Latin name we know today, *Calendula officinalis*, with *calendae* referring to the calendar.

Calendula is a readily self-seeding annual. One plant from the herb farmer will result in many more the following year. To contain them, it's best to cut off the spent flower heads before they dry, but if you have a garden like mine that chooses its own borders, you and calendula will get along just fine. The seeds are very unusual in appearance. When I first started making soap with calendula, I didn't carefully comb through the petals, and the first time I saw a seed, I was sure it was a small grub or worm. It was a huge relief to find that it was a seed, but not exactly the look I was going for with the soap.

Here on the farm, the petals are used in soapmaking and bathing herbs; the whole flowers are infused in oil for various preparations such as balms and lotions; and everything else (including the flowers I pulled the petals from) goes into the small (2-quart, or 2 L) distiller to produce a glorious hydrosol with just the tiniest bit of essential oil.

The resin that makes these flowers so sticky is full of great skin-loving medicinal properties. Antiseptic and anti-inflammatory, calendula has skin-soothing abilities that are hard to beat. Composed of carotenoids, flavonoids, and essential oils, it's also antimicrobial, antiviral, antifungal, and astringent while still being gentle. Calendula can make an amazing difference on stubborn rashes or just about any skin problem or irritation, even sometimes those that have been unresponsive to a doctor's attention. It has been found to be more effective than traditional allopathic treatment for radiation burns and is wonderful for sunburn. Eczema sufferers often find relief using an infused oil, either plain or made into a loose salve or lotion.

The gentle healing from this herb can be felt from as simple a remedy as a tea used as a wash or gargled for a sore throat and/or gums. For the sensitive skin of the tiniest babe to the paper-thin skin of the elderly, calendula is deceptively powerful in its ability to help build collagen and encourage wound healing by stimulating the immune response with minimal scarring. It is one of the most common herbs used in natural baby care products, from soaps to lotion to oil.

Internally, via tea or tincture, calendula has historically been used to brighten the spirits. All of the wonderful things it can do externally can also apply to all of the mucous membranes in the body. In particular, it helps with sore gums, can be a great healer for peptic ulcers, assists in healing and controlling reflux, and even calms irritable bowel disease. Calendula has been used to stimulate menstruation, so it is not recommended for use by those who are pregnant or wish to become pregnant.

Externally, tea bags laid on the eyelids or an eyewash made of calendula tea is very effective on conjunctivitis. Soaking feet in a strong infusion can curb athlete's foot, and it is useful

for other fungal issues. It can even be useful for yeast infections.

There are many instances where calendula can be helpful in caring for pets and barnyard animals. The tea applied to or sprayed onto "hot spots" calms and heals them. On insect bites, cuts, scrapes, and scratches, calendula as a compress, poultice, salve, or spray is safe and effective. Not bad for a beautiful flower that will grow just about anywhere!

In 2008, the International Herb Association chose calendula as the Herb of the Year. This designation means that an herb is important for medicine, is edible, and is useful in crafting. Calendula meets all of the criteria with both hands tied behind its back.

Medicinal Benefits

» Reduces inflammation
» Kills viruses, microbes, fungi, and other pathogens
» Astringent
» Treats burns and skin issues
» Heals wounds and reduces scars
» Astringent

CALENDULA BATH TEA

A soothing bath treatment after a day in the sun or wind, this blend can be very helpful for all kinds of itchy rashes and skin soreness.

Ingredients

½ cup calendula
½ cup rose petals
¼ cup comfrey
¼ cup (20 g) oatmeal

Directions

Mix together well. Store in an airtight container. Use approximately ¼ cup (20 g) per bath. Place the mixture inside a muslin bag or put it into the center of a washcloth and secure the corners with a rubber band. Heat 1 quart (1 L) of water to boiling, remove from the heat, and place the bath herbs in the water while running a bath. Pour the tea and the tea bag into the bath just before climbing in. The tea bag can be used as a wash-cloth on dry, itchy skin.

Yield » 1½ cups, or 6 applications

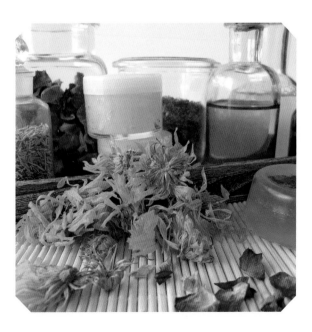

CALENDULA DIAPER RASH SALVE

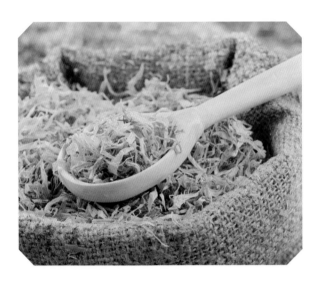

This gentle but effective salve is perfect for little bottoms.

Ingredients

⅔ cup (160 g) calendula-infused coconut oil
2 tablespoons (28 g) beeswax
¾ teaspoon zinc oxide powder

Directions

Coconut oil is solid at room temperature, so in order to infuse it with the calendula, low heat is required. It is also possible to warm it to liquefy, add the calendula, and leave it alone to infuse, but I'm never that patient. Infuse slowly for a few hours, and then strain very well so that there is no silt or grit. A coffee filter is slow, so it is the best method in this case.

Add the beeswax to half of the oil and heat slowly to melt the wax. When the wax is melted, add the zinc oxide and the remaining half of the coconut oil. Beat with a whisk or mixer until it is completely blended and starting to cool. Pour into jars and allow to set up. If it sets up too quickly to finish pouring into jars, a little heat will loosen it up again. Apply liberally to the skin.

Yield » ⅔ cup (160 g)

CALENDULA-LEMON GLUTEN-FREE SHORTBREAD WITH CALENDULA-LEMON POWDERED SUGAR

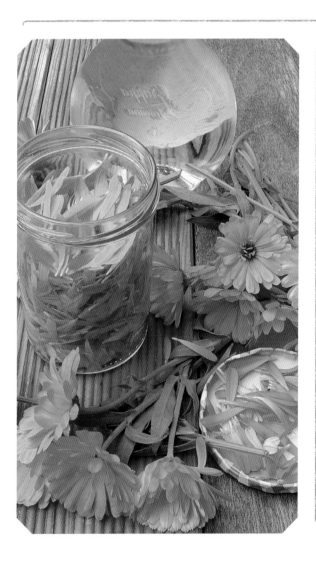

My favorite way to use calendula is to freeze a strong infusion in ice cube trays to have on hand for scrapes, for mouth sores, or (thawed) for burns. However, these cookies are a cheery way to bring calendula to a tea party or lunch. They pair beautifully with herbal tea, coffee, or a glass of milk.

Ingredients

For cookies:

½ cup (112 g) unsalted butter, softened

⅔ cup (132 g) sucanat or sugar

1 egg yolk

Zest from 1 or 2 lemons

1 teaspoon vanilla extract

½ cup (40 g) gluten-free oats

Petals from about 20 dried calendula blossoms

1 cup plus 2 tablespoons (178 g) superfine brown rice flour (measured first, then sifted)

¼ teaspoon salt

For powdered sugar:

Zest from 1 lemon

½ cup (60 g) powdered sugar, pulsed with petals from 6 calendula blossoms

Directions

To make the cookies: Cream together the butter, sugar, egg yolk, and lemon zest in a bowl. Add the vanilla and mix again.

In a spice grinder, pulse the oats and calendula blossoms until you get a fine flour. In a small bowl, mix together the oat/calendula flour, the sifted brown rice flour, and the salt, then add to the butter/sugar mixture. Mix completely. If dough is too wet, which can happen if your egg yolk is large, add just a little more sifted brown rice flour, 1 tablespoon (8 g) at a time, until you have a slightly stiff dough. It will be a little drier than drop-cookie dough.

Spoon out the dough onto a long sheet of waxed or parchment paper and form into a log. Roll up in the parchment and then gently continue to form the log for round or oval cookies, or square off each side to make square cookies. I make it squared by gently pressing each side against the countertop. Refrigerate for at least 1 hour.

Preheat the oven to 350°F (180°C, or gas mark 4). Line a baking sheet with parchment paper.

Remove the chilled dough from the refrigerator and slice off ¼-inch slices, placing them about 1 inch (2.5 cm) apart on the prepared baking sheet. Bake for about 12 minutes, or until the cookies are just slightly golden on the bottom. Allow the cookies to cool completely.

To make the powdered sugar: Mix together the lemon zest and sugar in a bowl and cover with a plate to allow flavors to infuse. Toss the completely cooled cookies in the powdered sugar mixture and serve. I like to garnish with a sprinkling of a few sunny calendula petals.

Yield » 3 dozen cookies

Source   Carey Jung, owner and creator at ApotheCarey Arts and Herbs, www.careyjung.com

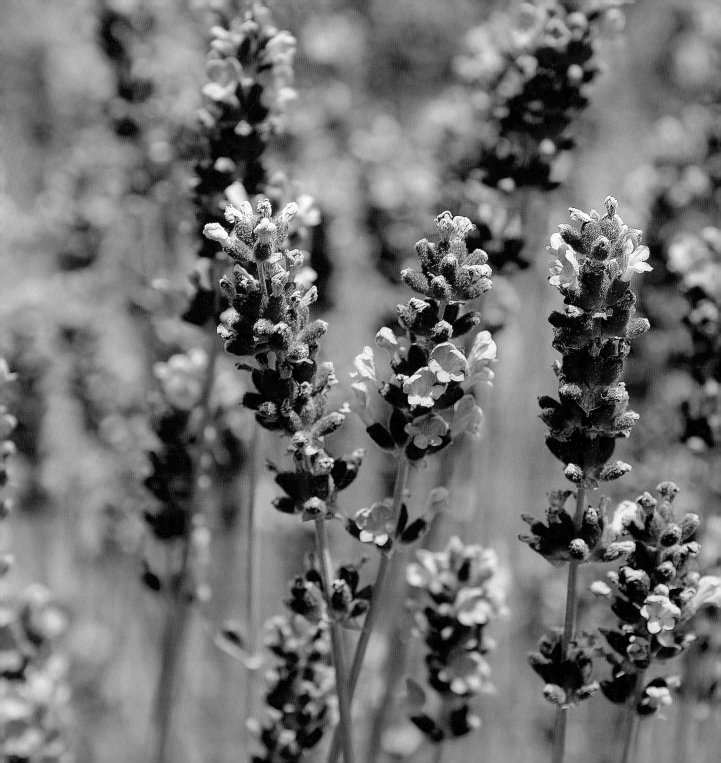

CHAPTER FOUR

Lavender

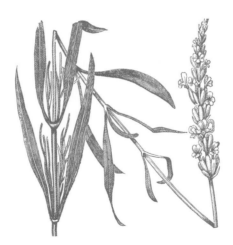

Lavandula spp.

Lamiaceae family

*L*AVENDER can be such a friend. With proper storage it stays useful and ready until you need it. Most people become familiar with the scent of lavender through the use of the essential oil in soaps, lotion, or candles. Getting its name from the Latin *lavare*, meaning "to wash," lavender clears the air, and because of that is sometimes added to ceremonial smudging blends where it becomes part of the incense. It is a clean, sometimes medicinal scent with floral notes. Some people love it right away. Others, like me, need to let it grow on them.

Early in my herbal learning days, I read an essay from a woman who always gave the gift of a pound (454 g) of dried lavender to celebrate a new home or a new marriage. She listed the myriad ways that the lavender could be used:

» Scattered under the rugs to keep a room fresh.

» Stuffed into small cloth bags and placed beneath seat cushions.

» Placed in a bowl near the door to be rubbed gently, releasing its scent before welcoming guests.

» Used in cooking and teas (sparingly).

» Made into sleep pillows.

» Added to baths, or made into strong tea to relieve skin rashes and irritations.

» Placed in closets and drawers to freshen and effectively repel moths.

At the time, I was dubious. Lavender conjured up thoughts of little old ladies and lace curtains. Time passed, and I came to love lavender almost above all others. I now have a row of 'Grosso,' a row of 'Hidcote,' and a patch of 'Provence.' These, along with 'Munstead,' are hardy varieties, and will survive most winters. Given shelter from the prevailing wind, or nestled up against a sun-warmed wall, most lavenders can grow in all but the very harshest areas. Lavender is one of my favorite herbs to distill in my small tabletop distiller. The flowers provide a tiny bit of essential oil and the hydrosol is a refreshing spray.

Lavender is a member of the large and helpful Labiatae family, with spikes in varying hues, from white, pale gray, and pink to pale lavender and the deepest purple, sailing above upright square stems. Native to the sun-drenched stony mountain slopes of the Mediterranean, it is the quintessential plant of the English country garden. The plants in early spring resemble rosemary, with flat, narrow, needlelike leaves.

The herb is mightily effective against moths. I visited a friend who had come into possession of the entire fleece of a shorn sheep. With a newborn, she didn't have much time to work on it, and when she opened it to show me, many small moths flew into the air. We scattered a few ounces of dried lavender buds in with the wool, and the next day the moths had moved on.

When my daughter was seven years old, school was a bit much for her. To help her with the stress, I made a small cat from black satin and stuffed it with lavender. It was about 4-inches (10 cm) tall, 2-inches (5 cm) wide, and perhaps 1-inch (2.5 cm) thick. She happily took it to school and kept it in her desk. A few weeks later I went to spend the morning assisting her teacher with a project, and was alarmed to walk in and find my daughter sitting with her head in her desk with the lid pulled down over her head. My alarm turned to amusement when I learned that it was between subjects and she was taking a short aromatherapy break. A couple of years ago I found the cat during a move. Fifteen years later, and the lavender still had plenty of scent when given a soft squeeze.

This use of lavender essential oil was the beginning of modern aromatherapy. The lavender plant has a relatively large quantity of essential oil compared to many other plants, so that we can use it in steams, infusions, compresses, and baths without necessarily needing to extract the potent oil. When I distill 2 quarts (2 L) of fresh chamomile flowers, I might obtain a single drop of the precious blue essential oil. Distilling

the same amount of fresh lavender flowers will likely result in ¾ teaspoon (3.5 ml) of essential oil. So as you might imagine, there's plenty of potent medicine in the fresh or dried flowers.

Lavender is best known as a remedy against insomnia, anxiety, and stress; it is thought to slow nervous system activity, allowing for a more restful sleep. Lavender calms a nervous stomach and may be helpful for relaxing and calming the entire gastrointestinal system. It contains antibacterial and antiviral abilities as well. Inhaling the steam produced from an infusion in water can help with upper respiratory issues, and headaches sometimes respond to the scent of the flower buds. On the skin, lavender can be soothing and healing for any sort of rash or burn, and many find relief from fungal infections and even eczema.

Medicinal Benefits

- » Aids sleep
- » Calms anxiety
- » Eases digestion
- » Kills bacteria, fungi, and viruses
- » Treats respiratory issues
- » Eases headaches
- » Soothes skin

LAVENDER LAUNDRY SACHETS

If you have access to small 3 x 4-inch (7.5 x 10 cm) muslin drawstring bags (often found in cooking supply stores), they work very well, but you can easily make your own. This is where those leftover socks come in handy.

Ingredients

¼ **cup lavender buds**

Directions

Add the lavender buds to muslin bag and tie the drawstring tightly, or if using a sock, pour the buds into the toe and knot the ankle of the sock. To use, simply toss the sachet into the dryer with the wet clothing. Clothes will come out smelling fresh and clean. This is especially nice for drying sheets, as the lavender scent lulls one gently to sleep. The sachet can be used at least three times.

Yield » 1 sachet

LAVENDER SPRAY

This can be used as an air freshener, a body spray, or a linen spray. It's easy and natural, and you'll find yourself using it a lot. The same method can be used for any number of essential oils or blends.

Ingredients

1 tablespoon (15 ml) vodka
3 ounces (90 ml) distilled water
30 drops lavender essential oil

Directions

In a 4-ounce (120 ml) spray bottle, mix all the ingredients. Keeping a spray in the fridge during the summer can make for a blessedly refreshing spritz when you take a gardening break and come in for a drink.

Yield » 4 ounces (120 ml)

SUNBURN OR WINDBURN VINEGAR

Because this is for external use and it is intended for use around the house, I generally opt for distilled vinegar because it's less expensive and the vinegar has no color of its own, so the herbs look pretty as they steep.

Ingredients

1 cup lavender buds

1 cup rose petals

Scant 1 quart (1 L) vinegar

Juice from 1 aloe leaf or 1 tablespoon (14 g) aloe gel per application

Directions

Combine the herbs in a 1-quart (1 L) jar. Fill the jar to the top with vinegar. Steep for 2 to 4 weeks. Strain. To use, combine the aloe gel with 3 ounces (90 ml) of the vinegar mixture in a spray bottle. Apply liberally to the weather-burned area for immediate relief.

Yield » 1 quart (1 L), 5 or 6 applications

LAVENDER AND FRANKINCENSE INCENSE

The term "loose incense" refers to incense that is not formed into cones or sticks, but is bits of botanical ingredients blended together to be sprinkled lightly on specially made charcoal blocks to smolder.

Ingredients

2 parts lavender buds

1 part crushed frankincense tears

Directions

Combine the herbs in a jar and use with an incense charcoal block.

Yield » As desired

LAVENDER SEASONING MIX

I think the most important thing about lavender and the one that took me the longest to master is that timing is everything when cutting the stems. The plants are ready for harvesting when the bottom third of the flower stem (known as a spike) is blooming. The magic window of time varies from garden to garden, depending on the rainfall, temperature variations, and ratio of sunny to cloudy days. You will need to check the plant daily because the spikes will not all be ready to harvest on the same day. I have only a dozen plants, and this small amount of plants makes selective harvesting possible. And what do I do with it? I cook with it! Many people know that herbs de Provence is a robust seasoning blend that uses lavender, but this blend has a stronger lavender flavor than that.

Ingredients

1 tablespoon lavender buds
1 teaspoon dried lemon thyme or garden thyme leaves
1 teaspoon minced dried chives
1 teaspoon dried parsley (Italian flat leaf is best)
1 teaspoon dried mint leaves
Black pepper to taste

Directions

Combine the herbs in a sealed jar for storage. Use to marinate eggplant, chicken, or pork by blending 2 tablespoons of the mix with ¼ cup (80 ml) oil and 1 tablespoon (15 ml) vinegar.

Yield » 2 tablespoons

Source   Marcy Lautanen-Raleigh, BackyardPatch.blogspot.com

LAVENDER-MARINATED CHICKEN AND SALAD WITH KIWI-LAVENDER VINAIGRETTE

For a refreshing summer salad, add lavender to a chicken marinade and combine it with kiwi in a vinaigrette for an unforgettable meal.

Ingredients

½ cup (120 ml) and 2 tablespoons (30 ml) olive oil, divided

¼ cup (40 g) finely chopped onion

2 tablespoons fresh lavender buds

2 fresh kiwi fruit, peeled and mashed

1 cup (235 ml) orange juice

4 chicken breasts

4 tablespoons (60 ml) fresh lime juice

Salt, to taste

4 cups (280 g) mixed salad greens

Directions

To make the chicken: In a small skillet, heat 2 tablespoons (30 ml) of the oil; add the onion and cook over medium-low heat until very soft, about 15 minutes. Remove from the heat and spoon into a large, shallow baking dish. Stir in the lavender, kiwi, and orange juice; whisk to combine. Place the chicken breasts in the marinade, turn to coat, cover, and set aside in refrigerator for 3 to 4 hours, turning occasionally.

Preheat the oven to 350°F (180°C, or gas mark 4). Lightly oil a baking pan.

Remove the chicken from the marinade and place in the prepared baking pan (do not discard the marinade). Cover with foil and bake for 45 to 50 minutes, or until the juices run clear and the chicken is cooked through. Remove from the oven and cool to room temperature. Slice into strips.

To make the dressing, bring the orange-lavender-kiwi marinade to a boil in a saucepan; lower the heat and simmer until reduced to about ½ cup (120 ml). Strain into a small bowl, discarding the solids. Whisk in the lime juice and remaining ½ cup (120 ml) olive oil, season with salt, and set aside to cool to room temperature.

At serving time, place 1 cup (70 g) of the salad greens in each of 4 salad bowls. Top with the sliced cooked chicken and drizzle with the lavender dressing.

Yield » 4 servings

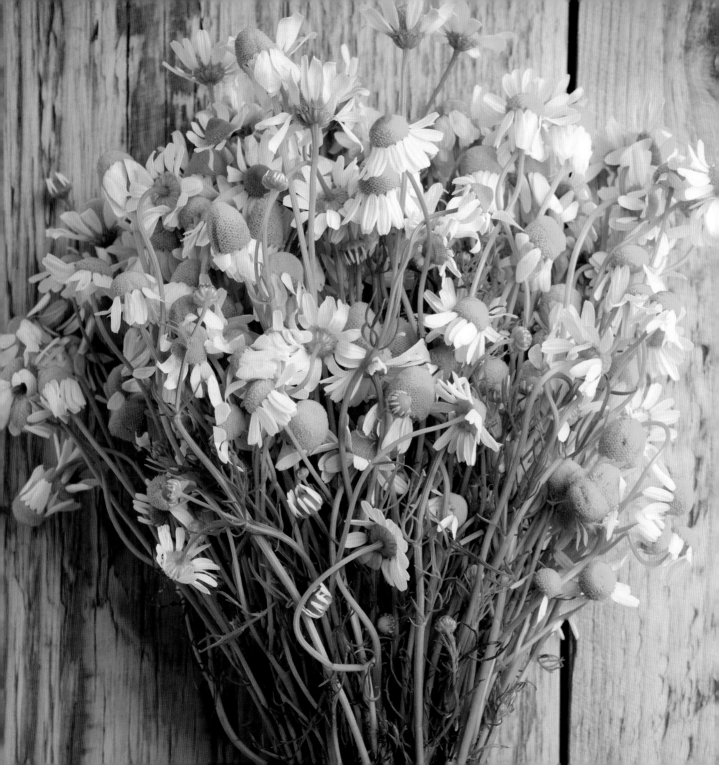

CHAPTER FIVE

Chamomile

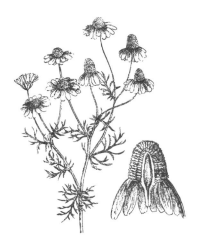

Matricaria recutita

Asteraceae family

CHAMOMILE was my first real experience with herbal medicine, and its sweet, light touch got my attention. There comes a time in all of our lives when we've allowed ourselves to become overextended. If we keep pushing, we find ourselves unable to put down the burdens and rest. I don't remember the circumstances that led to that state, but I certainly recall the blessed relief. I remember being on the verge of tears and under a lot of stress when someone finally suggested that I take a small break and have a cup of chamomile tea. I sat in an overstuffed chair, sipping the tea, and felt my shoulders release their tension. My neck relaxed. Soon I was asleep sitting up. That unassuming, tiny white daisy-like flower had worked her magic on me.

It is this quiet, unassuming quality that lends itself to being the perfect introduction to medicinal herbalism. We have become so accustomed to medicines that have strong, almost violent actions. They "knock us out" or "kick the flu," while herbs (with some exceptions) generally work in a more peaceful way. Hippocrates said, "Let food be thy medicine and medicine be thy food." Herbs are plants, plants are food, and one day they will be as common as apples and potatoes in the market. We're getting there.

The spring following that cup of chamomile tea, I set out to meet the herb on its own turf. After studying over the winter, I started looking. Sure enough, chamomile was everywhere. Armed with a cardboard box and a small shovel, I "rescued" a few square yards of it from a field being upon encroached by new development. Now, every summer there is plenty of chamomile, and there's something so meditative about sitting in a patch with a basket, plucking off the flower heads. I leave it in the large basket after harvesting. I keep it less than 1 inch (2.5 cm) deep, and each morning and evening I give the basket a gentle shake. It dries perfectly.

Matricaria recutita (also *Matricaria chamomilla*) is known as German or wild chamomile. This is the one often found in disturbed areas, in fields, and along roadsides. An annual, it spreads rapidly, with an upright, leggy growth habit. In my garden, it grows among tall daylilies, and competes with them for height. Sometimes it wins, but usually it falls over, proceeding to seed the yard. From this plant comes a sapphire blue essential oil that is very calming and often used in children's body care products.

Chamaemelum nobile, Roman, English, or garden chamomile, is a much more behaved plant, better suited for the garden. It grows closer to the ground and is sometimes used as a perennial ground cover, as it is resilient enough to put up with being walked on (sending up a soft, apple-like fragrance) and the occasional mowing. The essential oil obtained from this plant is pale yellow, and while it shares many properties with its blue cousin, it is more often used for skin care, relaxing properties, and a variety of aromatherapy applications.

Both of these plants are from the Asteraceae family, but it is important to note that they are completely different plants. Their appearance, scent, and many qualities and uses are very similar, but they are not varieties of the same plant. They are both growing in my backyard (although the German chamomile has now marched right out into the fields surrounding the yard), and it is very difficult to tell them apart. Many people are confused by the two, but fortunately drying the flowers and making tea from either plant will give you the same relaxing effect.

Both of these plants are native to Africa, Asia, and Europe and have become naturalized in the United States and most other temperate countries. There are records of use since ancient Egypt, and the sweet flowers and their stems and leaves were often used in medieval England as strewing herbs, or fragrant (sometimes pest-repelling) herbs that were used to compensate for some of the less than pleasant odors in homes where bathing was not common. They were strewn on the floors to release their fragrance when walked upon, a practice that persisted for hundreds of years. The word "chamomile" comes from the Greek *chamomaela*, or "ground apple." Pliny the Elder, an ancient Roman author and naturalist, described the plant as having the aroma of "apples or quinces." In Spain it has been known for centuries as mantazilla, meaning "little apple," and is used to flavor a light sherry that shares its name.

Chamomile is best known for its antiseptic, antispasmodic, relaxing, and anti-inflammatory properties. It is renowned as a tummy soother, popularized by Peter Rabbit's mother after his rough day with Mr. McGregor, and can help relieve menstrual cramping. It calms nerves and helps treat chest colds, sore throats, abscesses, and minor burns. A couple of freshly used chamomile tea bags laid upon the eyes is very soothing, and can help greatly with conjunctivitis. Healing for the skin and mucous membranes, it can be a wonderful addition to a bath tea.

Those allergic to ragweed should be cautious about chamomile, as the pollen present on the flowers may have an irritating effect for them.

Medicinal Benefits

- » Calming
- » Treats infection
- » Relieves cramping
- » Reduces inflammation

CHAMOMILE TINCTURE

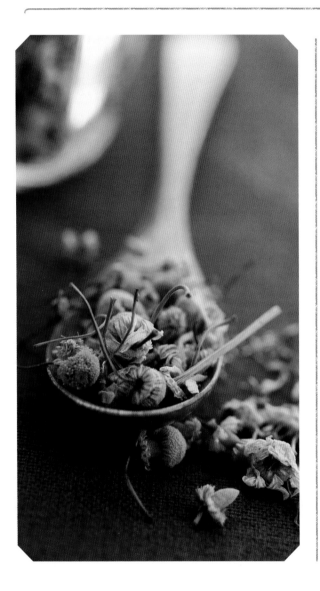

This has been a staple in my house for more than twenty years. As a wee one, my daughter was easily overstimulated and sensitive to sounds. We had tea parties with chamomile tea, but it wasn't always easy to get her to drink enough. I found that a few drops of tincture in any liquid calmed her, and later she came to reach for it in high school and college when first-day jitters or finals got to her.

Ingredients

Dried chamomile flowers
100 proof vodka

Directions

Fill any size jar loosely with dried flowers. Cover with the vodka. Place the lid on the jar and allow to steep for several weeks. One-half teaspoon is approximately equivalent to a strong cup of tea.

Yield » As desired

CHAMOMILE GELATIN

This soothing gelatin is a good choice for the sickroom when someone is restricted to clear liquids only.

Ingredients

1 (2.8-ounce, or 80 g) package apple-flavored gelatin

2 cups (470 ml) strong chamomile tea

Directions

Following the package directions for the gelatin, use chamomile tea in place of plain water. This is a great evening snack for kids, and just might be a brilliant idea to serve at stressful family gatherings.

Yield » 4 servings

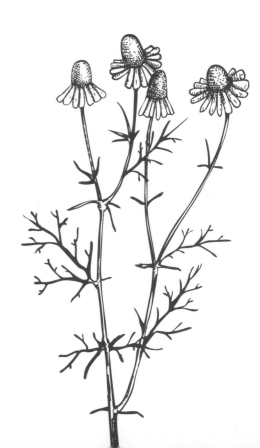

SLEEPY TEA

After studying chamomile and other soothing herbs, I have concocted the following tasty tea blend for a relaxing sleep. The reasons I chose these herbs is because chamomile encourages sleep and relaxation, hops is calming and helps with sleep, lemon balm and catnip relieve anxiety, and spearmint has a pleasing taste. I have shared this tea with friends and family. Everyone has commented about how helpful and relaxing it is.

Ingredients

½ cup dried chamomile
½ cup dried hops
½ cup dried lemon balm
½ cup dried catnip
½ cup dried spearmint

Directions

Combine the dried herbs together, store in 1-quart (1 L) jar, seal, and label. Use 1 heaping teaspoon in a tea ball to 1 cup (235 ml) of just-boiled water and steep for 5 minutes.

Yield » 2½ cups tea blend, 25 to 30 cups of tea

Source

Sandy Michelsen Kalispell, MT, www.etsy.com/shop/MontanaFolkRemedies

FACIAL STEAM

Essential oil of chamomile (and lavender, for that matter) is created through steam distillation. The steam carries miniscule particles of the essential oil up, away from the plant material, and in a facial treatment such as this, you're creating an instant hydrosol. Most people recognize hydrosols such as rose water or orange blossom water, but in fact steam such as this will carry along the essential oil from almost any oil-bearing plant.

Ingredients

1 cup dried chamomile flowers

Directions

Place the flowers in a large bowl. Pour boiling water into the bowl. After a few minutes of steeping, lean your face about 12 inches (30.5 cm) above the bowl and tent your head with a towel so that the steam from the bowl rises to your face. Breathing in the chamomile steam will also help sinuses and mucous membranes, especially in winter. A small handful of lavender added in is nice and healing in winter, as well.

Yield » 1 application

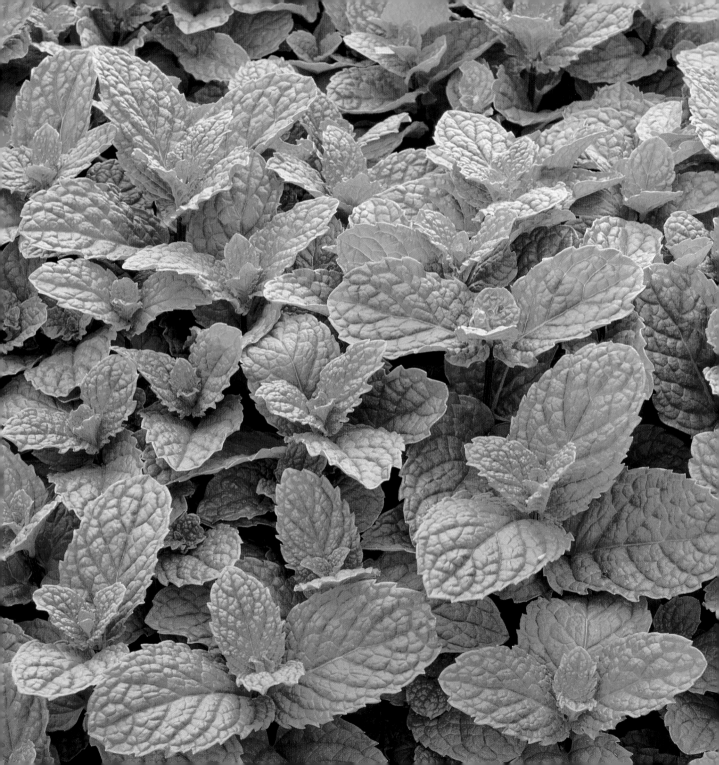

CHAPTER SIX

Mint

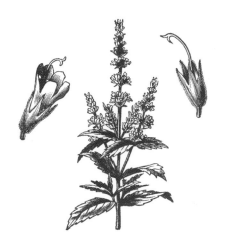

Mentha spp.

Labiatae (Lamiaceae) family

MY FIRST MEMORIES OF MINT revolve around the creek near where I grew up. It ran through a cow meadow, and the farmer didn't mind us kids playing there. Wild mint (*Mentha arvensis L.*) grew everywhere, along with the stinging nettles, wild mustards, forget-me-nots, jewelweed, burdock, and myriad other weeds, and we would often pick handfuls to take home and brew into sun tea. Often called "meadow mint," this variety is mild and tends more toward a spearmint taste than a peppermint. It is native to the United States.

The genus *Mentha* belongs to the plant family Labiatae, otherwise known as Lamiaceae. Other members of this family are rosemary, lavender, bergamot, basil, sage, and thyme. All of the plants in the Lamiaceae family have square stems, and often people say that the square stem means it is in the "mint family," but to be clearer, a mint must belong to the Lamiaceae family, but all Lamiaceaes are not mints.

Mint is named for a nymph in Greek mythology, Minthe. The god Pluto had fallen in love with Minthe, causing Persephone to become jealous. In a rage, she turned Minthe into a plant lying close to the ground. Pluto could do nothing to undo the spell, but gave Minthe the ability to smell sweeter with each footstep that trod upon her.

Throughout time, mint has been an honored plant. The oldest surviving medical text, the *Ebers Papyrus* (scrolls written in Egyptian hieroglyphics), is thought to have been written around 1500 BCE, but copied from other, earlier texts that went as far back as 3400 BCE, and there is mention made of peppermint for soothing the stomach.

Peppermint is mentioned in writings on the walls of the Temple of Horus in Egypt, and mint was accepted in payment of taxes in Egypt and Palestine during biblical times. As such, it was written in Luke (11.39): "You pay tithes of mint and rue . . . but you have no care for justice and love of God."

In ancient healing modalities from China and India (Ayurveda), physicians have used mint to treat poor digestion, coughs, cold, and fever, and as a general tonic. Ancient Romans and Greeks wore crowns of mint. Mint moved into Europe and Britain by the Romans, where it became popular as a strewing herb and an insect repellent. It was recorded in England by Nicholas Culpeper and Gerard. During the Victorian era, mint water was used to clean floors, was thought to remove negativity, and was hung in sickrooms.

We're all somewhat familiar with the use of mint in foods, beverages, mints, and gums, but we may not be aware of all the benefits offered. All of the mints have a wide variety of attributes, including analgesic, antimicrobial, antiseptic, antispasmodic, diaphoretic, digestive, repellant (insects), and stimulant properties. Besides freshening our breath when used in toothpaste, those antibacterial and anti-inflammatory properties kill bacteria and germs in the mouth, soothing gums and preventing decay. Simply chewing plain leaves of the mint plant can provide these benefits, too.

As an analgesic, mint is used in a cooling rub, and it is also used to clear the sinuses. Peppermint tea can be a real friend during a cold, especially when a cough and/or clogged sinuses are part of the deal. A few drops of mint essential oil dropped into hot water and inhaled (do not drink) can work wonders. Mints also have expectorant properties, helping to loosen and get rid of excess phlegm.

Many times I've read that peppermint can ease indigestion, but I always found it to make me feel worse. Recently while talking to herbalist Betty Pillsbury, she pointed out that peppermint relaxes muscles and esophageal sphincters, so that if reflux is an issue, it will be made worse. Spearmint will help settle the stomach without relaxing those sphincters, so it is a better choice for those with reflux. Peppermint is great for irritable bowel syndrome, cramps, bloating, and nausea.

Mint isn't usually considered for skin problems, but it can be incorporated into a good treatment for teenaged skin to prevent and heal pimples, acne, and blackheads. There is a fairly high amount of salicylic acid in the leaves, and the strong antioxidant, antibacterial, and anti-inflammatory properties make it an excellent choice for skin issues.

People who stand on their feet all day can find soothing relief from a cooling mint footbath that will also relieve itchy skin. In fact, many healing balms for skin use various mints to soothe, cool, and calm irritated skin. Mints are also antifungal, so it will help with athlete's foot, too.

Mint is also antispasmodic and relaxes the smooth muscles of the body. Mixed with some diuretic herbs, it makes a perfect PMS tea, curbing nausea, relaxing the muscles and preventing cramps, and even alleviating headaches.

Medicinal Benefits

» Eases digestion
» Treats cold and fever
» Combats cough
» Repels insects
» Relieves pain
» Kills microbes, bacteria, and other pathogens
» Eases cramping
» Induces sweating
» Stimulates
» Relieves inflammation
» Breaks up chest congestion and loosens mucus
» Clears up acne

MINT FLAVOR IN BAKED GOODS

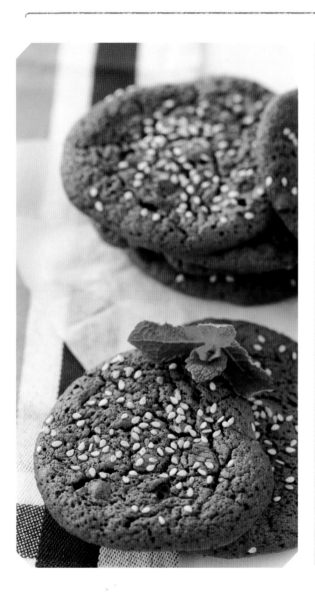

It's easy to add the zip of mint to any sort of baked treat by infusing the liquid or oil used with mint leaves.

» **Icing:** Infuse water or milk with mint before using.

» **Brownies:** Heat the oil with several mint leaves and cool before adding to the mix.

» **Cookies:** Add 1 to 2 teaspoons of dried mint leaves directly to the batter.

TABBOULEH SALAD

Here is a surprising and nutritious way to eat more mint, plus it's packed with vitamins!

Ingredients

1 cup (150 g) fine bulgur (cracked wheat)
3 cups (180 g) chopped fresh flat-leaf parsley
2 cups (192 g) chopped fresh mint
1 small onion, finely chopped
¼ cup (60 ml) lemon juice
½ cup (120 ml) olive oil
2 firm tomatoes, seeded and chopped
1 cucumber, peeled, seeded, and finely chopped
Salt and pepper, to taste

Directions

Prepare the bulgur by pouring boiling water over it and letting it cook without heat until soft (30 minutes). Drain and cool. Add all the other ingredients and mix together well.

Yield » 6 servings

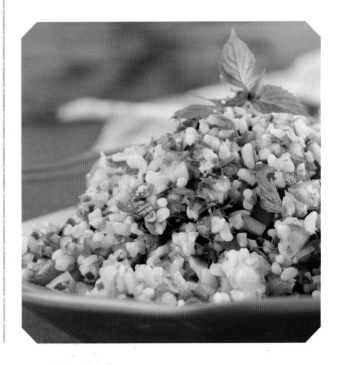

DOUBLE MINT TEA

Delicious anytime, this tea is particularly good after a heavy meal.

Ingredients

1 part dried spearmint
1 part dried peppermint

Directions

Blend the herbs together in a jar. Use a heaping teaspoon per cup (235 ml) of water. Steep for 5 minutes.

One of my favorite ways to enjoy this is by mixing it in equal proportions with black or orange pekoe tea (*Camellia sinensis*). It has the refreshing lift of mint with a little caffeine from the black tea, so it's a real pick-me-up in the middle of the afternoon.

Yield » As desired

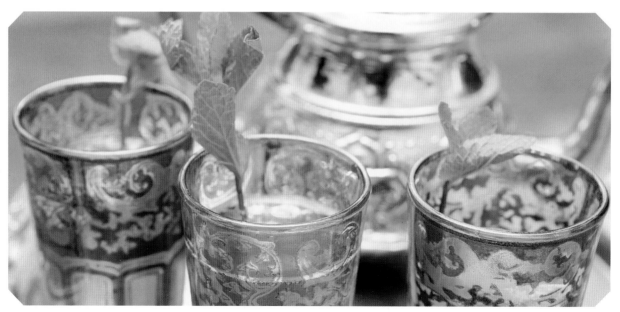

EASY AFTER-DINNER MINTS

Smooth, creamy, and rich, these mints are simple to make. I made them once for an open house when we had our herb shop. Instead of following the recipe (ask anyone, I'm notorious), I added three drops of essential oil instead of one. Please let me be a warning for others. They were some powerful mints! Stick to the recipe even though it seems like it can't possibly be enough. It is.

Ingredients

1 (1-pound, or 454 g) box 10X sugar
4 ounces (112 g) cream cheese, softened
One drop peppermint or spearmint essential oil
A few drops of green food coloring (optional)

Directions

In a bowl, work the ingredients together into a smooth, sweet, fragrant mass. It takes a little time and work, but it's worth it. This can be rolled into small balls and flattened slightly with the bottom of a glass, rolled out to ¼-inch (6 mm) thick and cut out with miniature cookie cutters, or pressed into candy molds. You can stop there, or you can dip half of them into melted dark chocolate to make them even more special.

Chill in the refrigerator for several hours before serving.

Depending on how large you make them, this makes a lot of mints. Fortunately, they freeze well and can be pulled out and enjoyed later!

Yield » About 100 (1-teaspoon, or 5 g) mints

NATURAL MINT TOOTHPASTE

This is a nice change from regular pastes and gels. I tried it a few times using essential oils, and couldn't get them to stay blended. That meant that sometimes I got no mint flavor while other times I got way more than seemed healthy. And so, I infused the oil! Repeatedly. The coconut oil in the recipe is triple infused with mint, and that fixed the problem for me. Coconut oil is great for the gums and teeth. It's often used in a healing technique called "oil pulling," where you swish the oil in your mouth for up to 20 minutes. I can't keep it going that long, but am happy to have coconut oil toothpaste!

Ingredients

½ cup (112 g) coconut oil
¾ cup (72 g) chopped mint, divided
½ cup (60 g) baking soda, divided

Directions

Combine the coconut oil and ¼ cup (24 g) of the mint in a saucepan and heat on low heat for 15 to 20 minutes. Strain. Repeat 2 more times, using the same coconut oil and ¼ cup (24 g) fresh mint.

To make a small batch of toothpaste, work together 1 tablespoon (14 g) of the infused coconut oil and 1 tablespoon (8 g) of the baking soda. Keep it in a small wide-mouthed jar by the sink. Repeat for new batches of toothpaste. Keeps teeth clean, slick, and fresh.

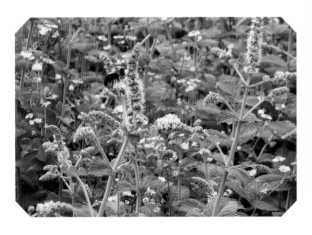

TIRED TOOTSIES TEA

Plain mint tea is a wonderful, cooling foot soak after one of those days when you've been on your feet all day and they feel as if they may be on fire. Adding a few other ingredients makes it superb.

Ingredients

1 cup (235 ml) apple cider vinegar
2 cups (470 ml) water
3 tablespoons dried peppermint leaves
2 tablespoons dried comfrey leaves
2 tablespoons dried lavender flowers
1 tablespoon (15 ml) olive oil

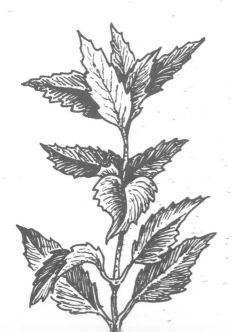

Directions

Combine the vinegar and water in a saucepan and bring to a boil over medium heat. Remove from the heat and add the herbs. Steep for 5 minutes. Strain and pour into a basin of warm water. Add the oil and stir to combine. Add some marbles or coarse salt if you have it. Place your feet in the basin and massage them on the salt or marbles.

The peppermint will cool. The comfrey will soothe. The lavender will help relax you. The vinegar will help slough off dead skin as you rub your feet on the marbles and/or salt. Finally, the oil will moisturize.

When you are ready, remove your feet from the bath and pat dry. Put on a pair of clean white cotton socks and relax. When you remove your socks, maybe even the next day if you decide to sleep in them, you will find your feet are soft and refreshed.

Yield » 1 footbath

Source   Maryanne Schwartz,
www.LancasterSoaps.com

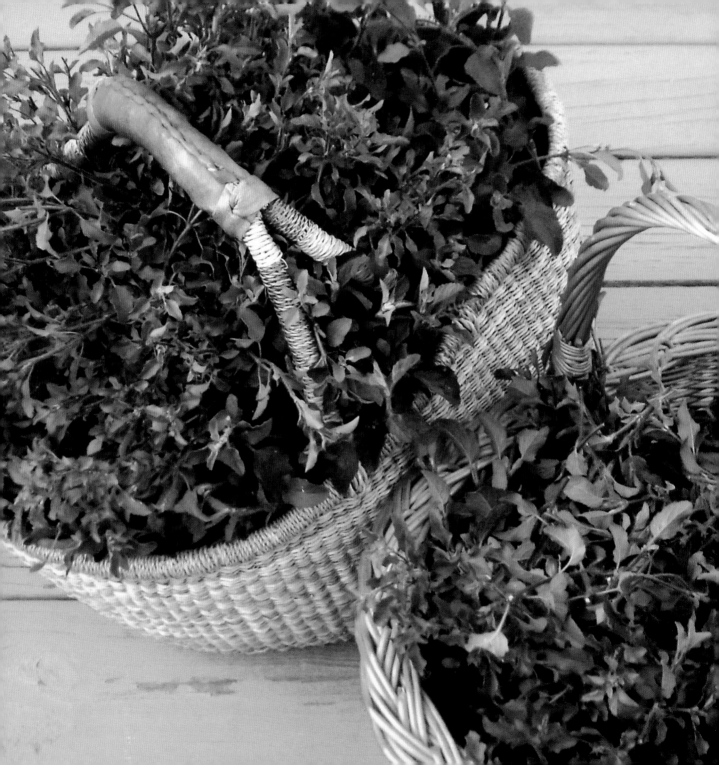

CHAPTER SEVEN

Basil

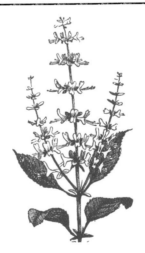

Ocimum spp.

Lamiaceae family

As with almost any very popular herb, there are many varieties. I was introduced to basil relatively late in life (mid-thirties) and have never looked back. I've yet to taste a basil I didn't like, and medicinally they are full of healthy benefits.

Holy basil, also known as tulsi, is one of my favorite varieties. It is no exaggeration to suggest that it saved my sanity, and quite possibly my life. During a long, brutal, seemingly endless stint as the primary caretaker for a terminally ill sibling, I learned that holy basil seems to have an effect on the way the body handles stress, reducing cortisol production and the resulting belly fat. I started doing more research into the herb, and realized it might just be what was needed for the stress and grief of caregiving.

It just so happened that I had grown a lovely, lush plant the previous summer on a whim. Not being sure what to do with it other than use it as a tea ingredient, I made most of the plant into a tincture. There are quite a few jars of tinctured herbs around here that may come in handy someday. Preserving them in alcohol keeps them available for many years.

My own personal experience with this plant is nothing short of miraculous. The stress and depression of my living situation was so severe that often while writing or working, I'd suddenly realize that there were tears rolling down my cheeks. Keeping it together was rough. However, after a single dose of the holy basil, it was as if the clouds parted. Nothing really changed except my point of view. I took it every day for the next couple of years. Now I am never without it. My friendly neighborhood herb farmer starts a whole flat for me each year and holy basil has a revered place in the garden. It did not help me lose any weight, but it had a profound effect on my stress management.

There are so many beautiful and tasty culinary varieties, including 'Opal', 'Genovese', 'Thai', 'Cinnamon', 'Licorice', 'Lemon', and 'Purple Ruffles'. The leaves can vary from tiny on the 'Spicy Globe' or 'Fino Verde' plants to large on the 'Lettuce Leaf' or 'Mammoth' varieties. I recently grew 'Lime' basil and found it to be delicious with fish, chicken, cheese, and tomatoes, as well as an unusual and welcome tea ingredient. My favorite all-around basil for summer cooking is 'Greek Columnar' basil. It grows on long straight stems, making harvesting very easy, and it never bolts because it is propagated only from cuttings. Because it doesn't bloom, the leaves are perfect from June until frost and I don't have to run out every couple of days to make sure it doesn't go to flower. Once an herb blooms (generally speaking), the flavor is not as delicious, and in herbs in which I prefer the leaf to the flower, keeping them from bolting can become almost a full-time job. It isn't quite as tender as the more typical sweet basils, but I'll sacrifice that for the convenience.

Basil does not dry well, meaning that its flavor, color, and components are not retained. It can be frozen: Process it into a paste with some olive oil and then freeze the paste into ice cubes. A cube or two can easily be pulled out to add to soups, stews, and pasta dishes in the middle of winter when you're longing for that fresh flavor. These days, it is fairly easy to find fresh basil in the produce section at the grocery store, so don't bother with the dried stuff.

The culinary basils are commonly thought of as a group known as sweet basil, and the most common of them is *Ocimum basilicum*. All of them impart vast health benefits, too. Best known for combating inflammation, basil is useful in conditions ranging from rheumatoid arthritis to inflamed bowels. Inflammation can occur in all parts of the body, and plants that combat it are our first and most important line of defense. More and more we are learning that inflammation is the basis of the serious diseases that degrade and end our lives. Heart disease, diabetes, possibly cancer, and all of the truly damaging diseases start out with inflammation somewhere. Thus, fighting inflammation is a top priority.

Many varieties of basil have a cinnamon note as a scent or flavor. These contain cinnamanic acid, which may help with high blood sugar, poor circulation, and respiratory ailments. Basil is also rich in antioxidants that combat aging and support the immune system. A simple tea made from basil can combat stress, help with upper respiratory illnesses, battle headaches, calm the stomach, and improve digestion. Basil is widely used to help reduce fevers. In Ayurvedic medicine, it is considered a general tonic and is used quite a bit for depression, headaches, digestive issues, arthritis, and toothache. Natural healing modalities all over the world have relied heavily on basil for thousands of years. Because it's such a tasty addition to the diet, it's easy enough to give it a chance to do its stuff.

Medicinal Benefits

» Reduces inflammation
» Reduces high blood sugar
» Promotes circulation
» Treats respiratory ailments
» Combats aging
» Supports the immune system
» Combats stress
» Improves digestion
» Combats headaches
» Reduces fever
» Eases depression

CUP OF KINDNESS TEA

This blend is formulated for the middle of winter, to help push the gray clouds away while supporting the immune system with virus-busting herbs. It can really help make a bad day better, and it tastes good, too.

Ingredients

½ cup dried holy basil
¼ cup dried rose petals
¼ cup dried lemon balm
¼ cup dried elderberries
2 tablespoons finely minced
   crystallized ginger

Directions

Blend all the ingredients well and store in an airtight container. Use 1 heaping teaspoon per cup (235 ml) of water. This can be drunk several times a day.

Yield » 48 cups (12 ℓ)

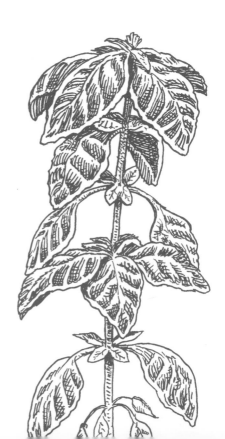

TOMATO-BASIL SALAD

There is nothing quite as refreshing on a warm summer day as fresh tomatoes with basil.

Ingredients

5 ripe tomatoes, cut into wedges
1 red onion, chopped
1 bell pepper, chopped (any color)
½ cup (20 g) chopped fresh basil
Freshly ground pepper
Oil and vinegar salad dressing

Directions

In a large bowl, combine the tomatoes, onion, bell pepper, and basil. Add ground pepper and mix well. Allow to set, refrigerated, for 1 hour.

Add your favorite oil and vinegar salad dressing, just enough to coat the vegetables. The amount may vary, depending on the juiciness of the tomatoes; start with ¼ cup (60 ml). Let this set in the refrigerator for another 2 hours for the flavors to meld.

To make this salad into an awesome hot-weather pasta dish, cook a pound (454 g) of pasta. I like rotini or fusilli to hold on to a little of the dressing, but choose your own favorite. While the pasta is hot, fold in ½ pound (226 g) cubed fresh mozzarella cheese. Mix in the salad and serve with a crusty bread for a simple rustic meal that doesn't take much time, and the leftovers are even better the next day.

Yield » 6 servings

TOMATO-BASIL QUICHE

This quiche is delicious as an appetizer or main course.

Ingredients

1 (9-inch, or 23 cm) pie crust, unbaked

¾ pound (340 g) Swiss cheese

12 medium eggs

1 pint (470 ml) half-and-half

½ teaspoon ground nutmeg

Pinch of cayenne pepper

2 teaspoons chopped fresh basil or 1 teaspoon dried, plus more for sprinkling

Freshly ground black pepper

1 tomato, sliced

Directions

Preheat the oven to 350°F (180°C, or gas mark 4).

Line a 9-inch (23 cm) pie pan with the crust. Grate the cheese into the crust. Put the eggs in a large bowl and beat with a wire whisk. Add the half-and-half, nutmeg, cayenne, basil, and pepper. Whisk again. Pour into the crust. Carefully lay the tomato slices on top of the egg mixture. Sprinkle with additional basil.

Bake until a knife inserted into the center comes out clean, about 45 minutes. Let stand for 5 minutes, and cut into wedges.

Yield » 8 servings

THAI BASIL SIMPLE SYRUP

This syrup may be used to drizzle over summer fruit such as strawberries, watermelon, or peaches and can also be a sweetener for iced or hot tea.

Ingredients

1 cup (200 g) sugar
1 cup (235 ml) water
½ cup (20 g) torn fresh Thai basil leaves, along with a few blossoms

Directions

Bring the sugar and water to a gentle boil in a small pot on the stove. Add the Thai basil and turn off the heat. Let the Thai basil sit in the syrup for about an hour minimum.

Remove the Thai basil and either use the syrup right away or refrigerate.

Yield » 1 cup (235 ml)

Source
Michele Brown, Possum Creek Herb Farm, www.possumcreekherb.com

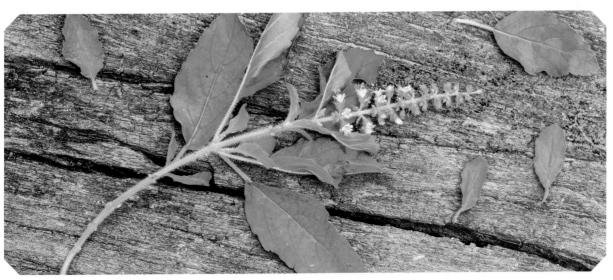

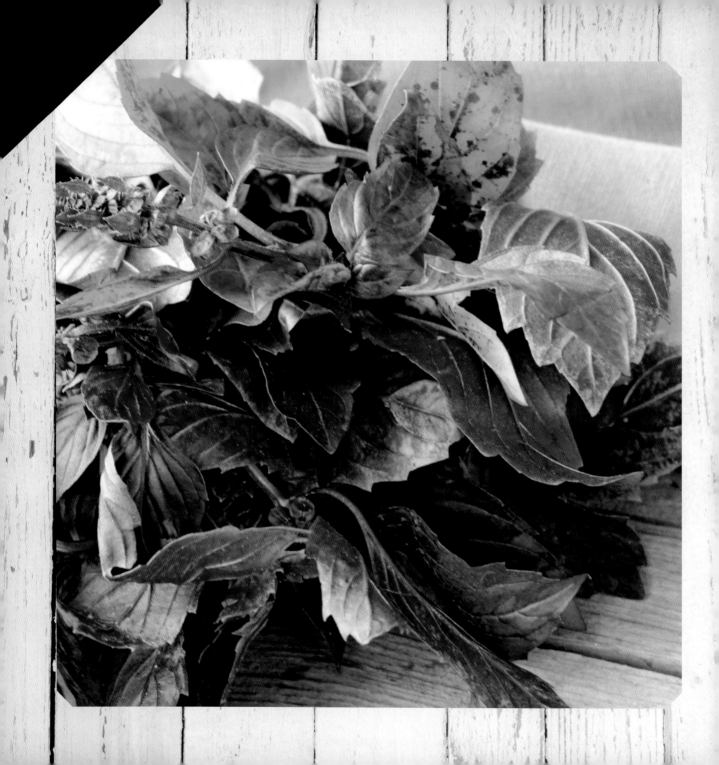

PURPLE BASIL VINEGAR

Vinegar made with one of the purple basils is a real stunner. The jewel tone of the plant infuses into the vinegar as does the flavor and can then be incorporated into some interesting salad dressings. It will turn a creamy dressing pink, and mixed with oil it retains that ruby color. In addition to the flavor, vinegar will take on the vitamins and minerals we so value in basil, as well as most of the other medicinal benefits. Any of the purple basils can be used, and if the color is not of interest to you, use any basil at all. Choose a mild, clear vinegar for this so that the color and flavor come through without being muddled. There are several choices, but please don't use distilled vinegar. It is more cleaning fluid than food.

Ingredients

1 quart (1 L) white wine vinegar
1 cup (40 g) clean, dry purple basil leaves

Directions

If the bottle of vinegar that you purchase is smaller than a quart (1 L), it isn't that important. In my own kitchen, I pick a large handful of leaves, fill a jar about half full with them, and then fill the jar with vinegar. Because I rarely throw away a jar, it could be anywhere from ½ cup (120 ml) to 2 quarts (2 L).

The vinegar will be pink within a few hours, but leave it for a few weeks to fully develop. Strain it, and pour into any clear, clean bottles you'd like. Do not store this in sunlight, or it will fade. I know it's tempting to show off that color, but keep it in the cupboard until it's time to bring it out for use.

Yield » 1 quart (1 L)

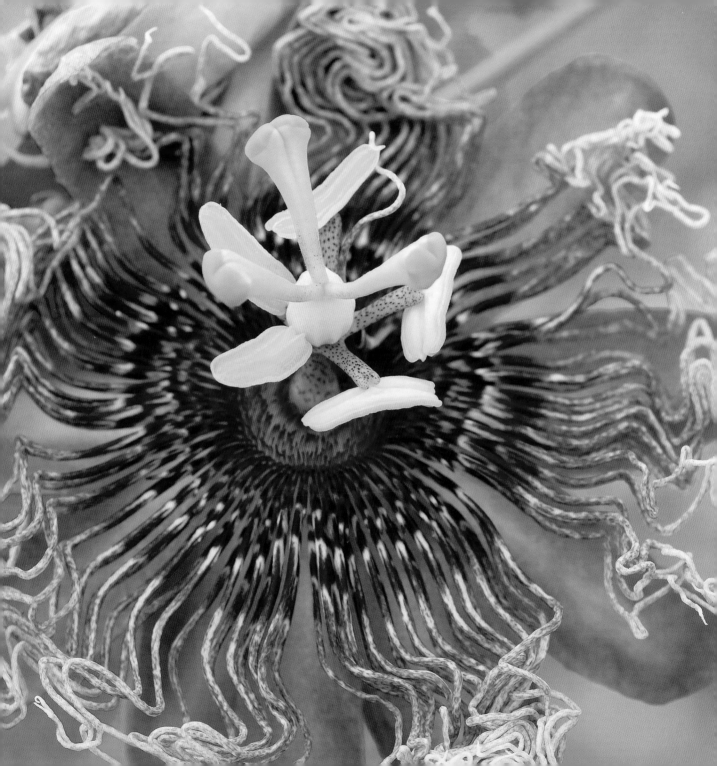

CHAPTER EIGHT

Passionflower

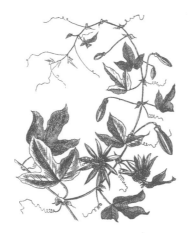

Passiflora spp.

Passifloraceae family

PASSIONFLOWER'S VERY UNUSUAL blooms do not appear to possibly be real. The short stems on the flower itself do not lend themselves well to cut flower arrangements, so you would almost never see them as such. At my house, I can't resist bringing them inside. After chasing away any of the ants that love them, I simply float them in a shallow dish of water so that they may emit their lovely fragrance and allow me to gaze upon them for a few days. In a tincture, the whole flowers, leaves, and tendrils turn a ghostly white, and that jar has frightened more than one visitor!

There are more than 200 species of passionflower in the world. Varying shades of purple, reds, creams, and white festoon the vines. The center corona can be made up of straight or wavy spikes that can vary in color as well. The wild *Passiflora incarnata* is the Tennessee state flower, and is mostly used for food and medicine. Sometimes called *maypop* (perhaps because of the way the stems pop out of the ground in May), it produces a fruit that in my zone (7) has yet to ever ripen sufficiently to eat. The unripe fruit and the outer rind of the fruit (even when ripe) contains cyanide precursors, of which the smell can sometimes be present, and should not be eaten. The inside of the fruit, bearing many seeds, is said to be delicious, but I cannot personally attest to that. Not yet, anyway.

Although the name *passionflower* has a sexy connotation, and has on occasion been thought of as an aphrodisiac, the name comes from symbolism derived from the Christian religion. Its original name, given by the Cherokees, is ocoee, leading to the Ocoee River and Ocoee River Valley in Tennessee to be named after the plant. Spanish explorers in South America "discovered" passionflower and named it, seeing religious symbols in the leaves (hands of Christ's persecutors), corona (crown of thorns), and five stamens (wounds). Explorers in Peru saw these signs and took them as a blessing on their venture.

Passionflower possesses woody stems that grow at an amazing rate. Mine dies back to the ground every year, but the stems reach 20 to 30 feet (6 to 9 m) by the end of summer. The leaves are alternate and palmate (resembling hands), almost always with three lobes. The leaves are distinctive and easily recognizable once you've seen them. Prodigious numbers of beautiful curly tendrils help the vine grow and climb. It can be quite invasive. It prefers partial shade, but full sun does not seem to be holding it back. Each year there are twice as many stems leaping from the ground, sprawling along the split-rail fence, and climbing up the tall Jerusalem artichoke stalks that grow nearby. If you choose to plant some passionflower vines, do heed this warning. It requires a lot of space and moving or removing it will require vigilance.

One of the most important qualities of passionflower is its ability to calm a busy mind. People who have trouble sleeping because they go around and around with circular thinking, dwelling on problems, worrying, and fretting, will find solace in passionflower.

Promising research has been done that indicates that passionflower can be as effective on anxiety as the pharmaceutical diazepam without the harmful addictive side effects. In fact, passionflower may be very helpful in reducing symptoms and difficulty with withdrawal and addiction to alcohol, nicotine, and other drugs. Most of the research focuses on using alcohol extracts of the plant, which is contraindicated for use with alcohol addiction, but in that case the infusion or tea is made with water. Using passionflower in conjunction with sedative medications is not recommended because it may increase the action too much. It is a uterine stimulant, so should be avoided during pregnancy.

Passionflower is good for muscle spasms. It may not be the first thing you'd think of when your back tightens up, but perhaps it should be.

This herb also calms the central nervous system. Levels of neurotransmitters, especially GABA (gamma-aminobutyric acid), are increased, slowing the activity of nerve cells and allowing mental stimulation to decrease and relaxation to take place. Because of this activity on calming the nerves, passionflower can be quite helpful in cases of shingles, especially in conjunction with herbs such as St. John's wort and lemon balm, when used both internally and externally. It has been used for tension and fatigue, and some herbalists feel that it can be of assistance in lowering blood pressure. As with many herbs, it can thin the blood somewhat. There have been reports of its use for hyperactivity in children with varying degrees of success.

This mild but effective sedative and relaxant herb may also be of assistance for asthma and coughs. Native Americans used the macerated leaves as a poultice on bruises and injuries and used the vines as a tea. Currently, all aerial parts are used medicinally.

Medicinal Benefits

» Aids sleep

» Calms anxiety

» Reduces withdrawal symptoms

» Eases back spasms

» Lowers blood pressure

» Alleviates cough and asthma

CALM CANDY

The herbs in this candy help relieve anxiety, stress, and overexcitement.

Ingredients

1½ cups (355 ml) water

¼ cup fresh passionflower

¼ cup fresh lemon balm

¼ cup fresh chamomile

Juice and zest of 2 lemons

Unsalted butter

3 cups (600 g) sugar

½ cup (160 g) corn syrup or honey (if using honey, the candy will probably remain sticky)

Confectioners' sugar or cornstarch, for sprinkling

Directions

Combine the water, herbs, and lemon juice and zest in a large saucepan over medium-low heat. Simmer to reduce the liquid to 1 cup (235 ml). Meanwhile, butter a baking dish.

Add the sugar and corn syrup and stir until the sugar dissolves. Clip a candy thermometer to the side of the pan. Increase the heat, bring to a boil, and boil to 300°F (150°C), with as little stirring as possible. Remove from the heat and pour the hot mixture into the baking dish. Let cool.

As soon as it can be handled, cut into pieces and sprinkle with confectioners' sugar or corn-starch to keep the pieces from sticking together. Alternatively, pour onto a butter baking sheet to ¼-inch (6 mm) thick, and break into pieces when cooled.

Yield » 1 pound (454 g)

BEDTIME TEA

This nighttime tea is a good choice for days when everyone is overly tired or having trouble winding down. You can use the tea in place of water when making gelatin for a bedtime dessert.

Ingredients

1 cup (235 ml) water
1 teaspoon passionflower
1 teaspoon chamomile
1 teaspoon lemon balm

Directions Combine the water and herbs in a saucepan and bring to a simmer. Remove from the heat and let steep.

Yield » 1 cup (235 ml)

BATH FOR RESTFUL SLEEP

A nice warm bath infused with these ingredients helps soothe the cares of the day and their physical manifestations.

Ingredients

¼ cup dried passionflower
¼ cup oat straw
¼ cup (90 g) Epsom salts
Boiling water

Directions Place the ingredients into a muslin bag or tie into the center of a washcloth. Make sure the herbs have enough space to infuse easily. Place in a 2-quart (2 L) pitcher (rigid plastic is fine). Pour boiling water over the herbs and steep for 10 to 15 minutes while running a bath.

Pour the steeped bath tea and packet into the tub. Soak in a full tub. The magnesium in the Epsom salts makes a great addition to the antispasmodic, relaxing action of the herbs.

Yield » 1 application

NIGHTY-NIGHT ELIXIR

Most herbalists will tell you that it's best to make tinctures as single ingredients, and blend them later. That way, if you need one of them without any of the other herbs, you have it. Once you've blended them, you're stuck with the blend. Usually I agree with that, but sometimes I break the "rules." A friend of mine was having a terrible time getting to sleep, and I wanted to make him something that didn't involve a lot of liquids before going to bed. At the same time, I was pretty broke financially at the time, so I got a very nice relaxing tea blend from Susanna Reppert at the Rosemary House, and used it to make an elixir. I've tinkered with it a little over the years, and it has helped just about everyone except the person it was made for. Oh well. You can't win them all.

Ingredients

½ cup passionflower
¼ cup chamomile
¼ cup lemon balm
¼ cup valerian root
2 tablespoons skullcap
2 tablespoons motherwort
1 tablespoon lavender buds
4 ounces (112 g) honey
1 to 1½ cups (235 to 355 ml) vodka

Directions

Place all the botanicals in a pint (470 ml) jar. Pour the honey over them and stir to coat them. Add vodka until the jar is filled and the plants are submerged.

This mixture needs to age for a month. When it's finished, strain out the herbs and use about 1 tablespoon (15 ml) of the elixir about 30 minutes before bed.

Yield » About 1½ cups (355 ml)

PASSIONFLOWER TEA

Passionflower makes a great tea for relaxing mind and body without making you feel drowsy, so it is a great tea to drink during the day to help you focus.

Ingredients

2 teaspoons passionflower leaf, vine, and flower
1 cup (235 ml) boiling water
Honey (optional)

Directions

Add the herb to the water and steep for 15 minutes. Sweeten with honey, if desired.

Yield » 1 cup (235 ml)

SLEEPYTIME TEA

Mixed with other herbs, passionflower is wonderful for a sleepytime tea. This is one of my favorites for having in the evening before bedtime. This blend calms the mind, relaxes the nerves, and lulls you to sleep, encouraging a night of restful sleep.

Ingredients

1 cup dried passionflower leaf, vine, and flower
½ cup milky oats
¼ cup lemon balm leaves
¼ cup chamomile flowers
2 tablespoons California poppy aerial parts
2 tablespoons motherwort leaves
1 tablespoon catnip leaves

Directions

Combine the ingredients together and store in a glass jar. To use, add 1 tablespoon to 1 cup (235 ml) of boiling water. Allow to steep for 15 to 20 minutes. This is best enjoyed during or after a warm bath.

Yield » 2¼ cups

Source for both recipes Kristine Brown, www.herbalrootszine.com

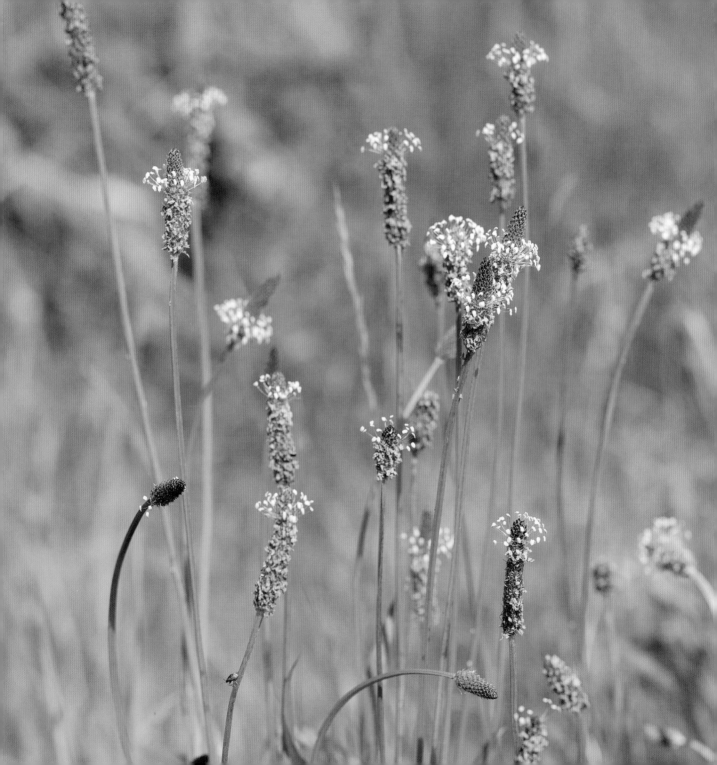

CHAPTER NINE

Plantain

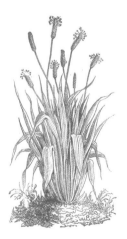

Plantago major and *Plantago lanceolata*

Plantaginaceae family

Bring plantain up in discussion with a room full of herb enthusiasts and you'll be surprised at how much excitement you'll find for a lowly lawn weed that millions of people spend a fortune trying to eradicate. The two common varieties are *P. major* and *P. lanceolata*, and they have many nicknames: ribwort, narrowleaf plantain, English plantain, buckhorn plantain, lanceleaf plantain, ribgrass, and many more. In my childhood they were "rabbit's ears" and I've heard people call them "pig ears" and "lawn lettuce," among others.

Plantain grows all around the globe. It is thought that it was naturalized in part through contamination of grain destined for seeding during harvest and sown right along with the grain in new fields in new places.

There are more than 200 species of plantain, but I will focus on these two, the best known, easiest to find, and most used. They are so interchangeable that other than a description, I will not differentiate between *P. major* and *P. lanceolata*. They are perennial weeds growing from a small rosette that becomes quite lush. In semishaded protected places, I've seen the leaves of both become more than 6 inches (15.2 cm) in length, and *P. major* nearly as wide. *P. lanceolata* can get over a foot (30.5 cm) long.

Usually about the day after you mow your lawn, their seed stalks (inflorescences) spring up 4 or 5 inches (10 or 12.5 cm), and *P. major* has long spikes of seeds while *P. lanceolata* bears shorter, cone-shaped seed heads on top of the thin, whiplike stems. In another day or two, delicate rings of tiny, creamy white flowers open on the spikes. At this point, your lawn looks pretty ragged. At least mine does. Between the plantain and the dandelions, I swear I can hear the neighbors groan when they stroll by.

This is another plant that can open your eyes to the miracle-like powers of herbs. Antibacterial, astringent, anti-inflammatory, antiseptic, demulcent, diuretic, expectorant, laxative, and refrigerant are just the beginning of the list of benefits from this plant. The leaves, seeds, and roots are all valued in medicine, and the leaves (particularly young, tender leaves) are a wonderful addition to salads or cooked as a vegetable similar to spinach; they contain lots of essential minerals, calcium, iron, potassium, and vitamins A, C, K, B$_1$, riboflavin, and carotenes with a relatively low amount of oxalic acid. Those dark green leaves are full of good health.

Plantain offers immediate relief for bee stings. Chop it or mash it and heat it briefly if you can. It will deter swelling and pain. Plantain contains aucubin, an antitoxin; in addition to pulling out the venom, it actually works to stop the venom's effects.

Plantain also contains allantoin, which promotes wound healing, speeds cell regeneration, and has emollient and soothing effects. Plantain is safe to eat or take internally, and that is very welcome news. It has styptic properties as well. Injuries to the entire digestive system can benefit from ingesting one of the many forms of plantain—as a tea, tincture, soup or broth, or vegetable.

The seed husks of plantain will, when wet, expand and exude mucilage, facilitating easier elimination of the bowels by swelling in the gut and acting as a bulk laxative while soothing irritation along the way. Commercially, seeds of *P. psyllium* are harvested specifically for this purpose, and the powdered seeds and husks are the main ingredient in Metamucil. *P. psyllium* has the highest percentage of mucilage, but the plantain seeds growing in your yard are quite adequate. *P. psyllium* will draw out moisture, which is helpful in moving the bowels.

The leaves are emollient, and are often used in teas, syrups, or tinctures for sinus congestion, coughs, all sorts of stomach complaints, middle ear infections, and more. The root is said to have been used for toothache and snakebite. Those two things sound very different unless you consider that in both cases, toxins need to be pulled out. Poultices are used for everything from splinters, sunburns, rashes, cuts, and scrapes to reports of old-time use on tumors.

In recent generations, the use of plantain has become mostly external. Salves, soaps, balms, and preparations of all kinds are readily available, and so we've stopped thinking of it as a food or an internal medicine. I think that's very sad, considering all it has to offer us.

Have plantain at the ready. Here are some simple ways to keep it on hand:

» Dry plantain leaves in summer to keep on hand. Lay on a screen in a cool, dark place. When completely dry, store in a sealed jar.

» Infuse olive oil with plantain leaves, fresh or dry. See page 90 for instructions. There are innumerable ways to use this oil: directly on the skin, mixed with vinegar for salad dressing, in balms, in the bath, or after a shower. You will wonder how you lived without it, especially if you live in an area with dry air.

» Make a strong infusion of plantain in water, and then freeze into ice cubes. Empty cubes into a storage container and keep frozen until ready to use.

» Steep some plantain vinegar. Use good-quality vinegar so that it can be used both internally and externally. Not distilled white, okay? Fill a jar loosely with fresh, clean plantain leaves. If you'd like to include some roots, that's fine too, but mostly leaves. Cover with vinegar and place a nonreactive lid on the container. Allow to steep indefinitely,

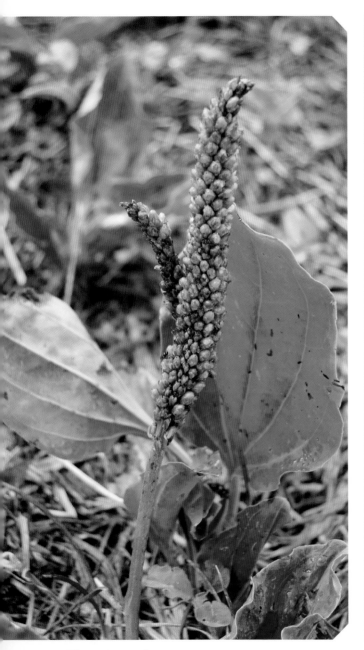

Plantago major

straining it when you're ready to use it. You might use the vinegar in a salad dressing, to spray on a sunburn, or to use as a hair or facial rinse to soothe and maintain a healthy pH balance. A spoonful of vinegar mixed with water or juice each day could be helpful with chronic bronchitis, sore throats, persistent coughs, and myriad digestive issues.

Medicinal Benefits

» Kills bacteria and other pathogens
» Tightens tissues
» Reduces inflammation
» Soothes mucous membranes
» Stimulates urination
» Loosens mucus
» Facilitates bowel movements
» Reduces body temperature
» Heals and soothes wounds and stings

FRIED PLANTAIN GREENS

Gather young leaves, no more than 4 inches (10 cm) in length.

Ingredients

3 tablespoons (45 ml) toasted sesame oil
1 scallion, minced
1 quart plantain leaves

Directions

Heat the oil in a frying pan over medium heat and add the scallion. After the scallion starts to soften, add the plantain leaves and cook, stirring often, just until they wilt slightly and are heated through.

Yield » 4 servings

PLANTAIN FIELD POULTICE

I often hear the phrase "spit poultice," and that's really what this is. In the case of a bee sting, mosquito or spider bite, nettle sting, or poison oak/ivy/sumac exposure, put a few leaves of plantain in your mouth and chew just long enough to break down the leaf structure and moisten so that it can mold to the wound or area. Rolling the leaves tightly in your hands or between your fingers will have the same effect, although the spit really does help hold it together.

PLANTAIN SKIN CARE

I love the skin-regenerating properties of plantain and use it extensively in my skin care line. It can be used as either an oil infusion or a water extract (decoction). The long-leafed variety in particular is easy to gather.

The easiest method for a do-it-yourselfer is to make a balm for chapped lips or skin. To do this, infuse your dried plantain in oil such as olive oil, sunflower oil, or almond oil. Mix your infused oil with cocoa butter and beeswax. The amounts should be about 60 percent infused oil, 20 percent cocoa butter and 20 percent beeswax. Or for a simplified recipe, try the following.

Ingredients

3 tablespoons (45 ml) plantain-infused oil
1 tablespoon (14 g) cocoa butter
1 tablespoon (14 g) beeswax

Directions

In a saucepan, heat all the ingredients gently over low heat until melted. Stir together and pour into tins. Let solidify before putting lids on the tins. If you want a balm that is less firm, use less beeswax.

Yield » 5 tablespoons (75 g)

Source
Dr. Cindy Jones, cosmetic scientist, herbalist, and owner of Sagescript Institute and Colorado Aromatics, www.sagescript.com

PLANTAIN TEA

Plantain tea has a decent taste alone, but it is excellent mixed with lemon balm. The mucilaginous properties of plantain also help ease an upset stomach.

Ingredients

1 teaspoon dried plantain leaf
1 teaspoon dried lemon balm leaf
1 cup boiling water (235 ml)

Directions

Combine the herbs in a tea ball. Pour boiling water over and let steep for 5 minutes. Drink.

Yield » 1 serving

Source
Dr. Cindy Jones, cosmetic scientist, herbalist, and owner of Sagescript Institute and Colorado Aromatics, www.sagescript.com

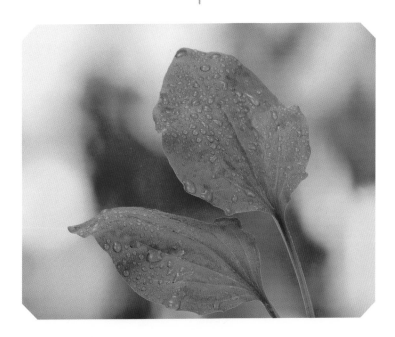

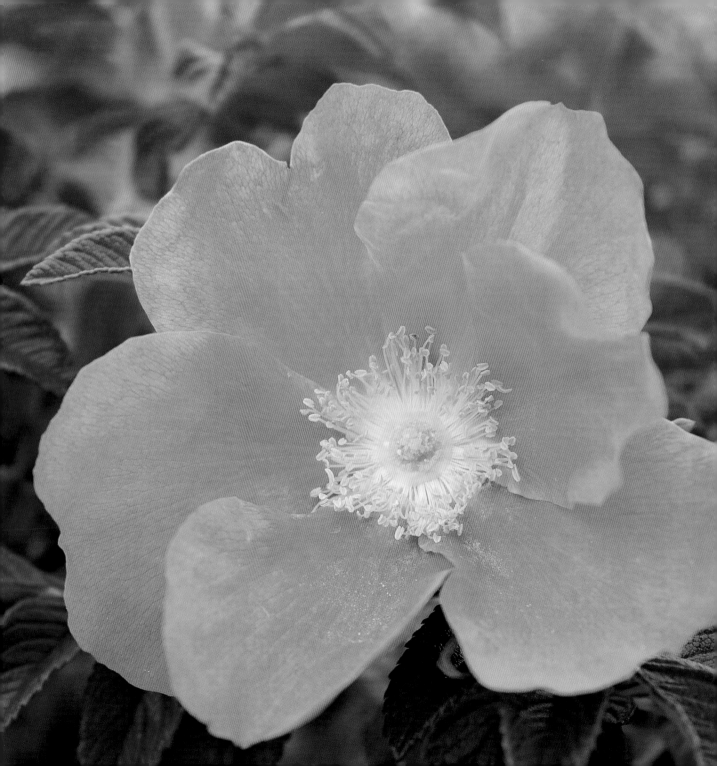

CHAPTER TEN

Rose

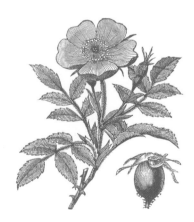

Rosa spp.

Rosaceae family

THE LORE concerning roses is extensive. The term *subrosa* came about in Roman times when a rose was hung upside down over the dinner table, signifying that the conversations held were to be kept confidential. A rose painted on a sign became the symbol for the medieval craft of apothecary. William Shakespeare often included references to roses in his writing. It is said that Cleopatra covered the floors of her palace knee-deep with rose petals to seduce Mark Antony, and the sails of her barge were soaked in rose water. The emperor Nero was so enamored of roses that he had an installation that spritzed rose water onto dinner guests during banquets, and the ceiling opened to drop rose petals onto the guests. Wild roses are a part of many Native American designs, and rose hips were a valuable food source for many tribes. In the Ojibwe language, the word for rose hips is *oginiiminagaawanzh*, which translates to "mother fruit from a small bush."

At various points in history, roses have been worn as crowns, scattered before royalty and brides, eaten, drunk, and even used in the mortar of buildings. Rare is a love potion or spell that does not include rose. Pliny the Elder listed more than thirty medicinal uses for rose during the first century AD. Roses have been cultivated and used for centuries.

The Rosaceae family is large and is very often aligned with the heart, both physically and emotionally. There are more than 10,000 rose species, varying from the small white multi-flora rose that scents the back roads and valleys near my home in early spring to the lovely cabbage roses such as Centifolia, Damask, Gallica, Cannina, and tea roses, and thousands in between. Roses come in many forms, sizes, colors, and even fragrances.

The volatile oil in rose (as well as more than 100 identified constituents—so far) has many healing properties; it is antidepressant, highly antioxidant, antispasmodic, aphrodisiac, astringent, antibacterial, antiviral, antiseptic, strongly anti-inflammatory, blood tonic, cleansing, cooling, digestive stimulant, expectorant, bile production stimulant, kidney tonic, and menstrual regulator, making this fragrant beauty a full-blown medicine cabinet on a stem.

Its astringent properties make rose a good addition to a tea or gargle for a sore throat. Antibacterial and antiviral, it can help fight infections of the intestinal tract. It is also a great support for the immune system, making it valuable in cases of cold or flu. Rose water has been used for many years for the skin, and the tea or a poultice of the leaves and petals can be a soothing and revitalizing facial. Rose petal vinegar relieves the pain of sunburn and makes a wonderful hair rinse as well as an intriguing ingredient for dressings or sauces, so be sure to infuse some petals in vinegar. Rose petal tea or

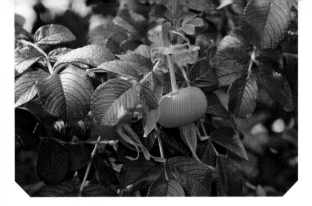

salve made from infusing petals in oil is great for rashes and dry, sore skin.

More than anything else, rose helps open the heart to hope. It relieves anxiety and is a cooling, calming tonic for the nerves. For people struggling with self-doubt, anxiety, or peri-menopause, rose will relieve the tension and support the organs that need to release the toxins these emotions throw into the bloodstream.

I have an entire hillside planted with *Rosa rugosa*. The first year or two there were goats living on the same hillside, and the flowers were kept a little too well manicured. Now goat-free, the deep green leaves burst forth in May followed by billows of magenta, pink, and white blossoms with a scent that nearly rolls my eyes back in my head. I gather as many as possible, feeling that the greater the fragrance, the stronger the medicine.

In the fall, I gather the plump rose hips for use in soap and syrups. The flavor is a bit sweeter after a frost, but I try to catch them while they are still plump so that I can peel the outer, usable part away easily from the dense interior ball of hairy seeds. The strips of the deep orange flesh, perfect for teas or syrup, are then dried and stored in a tightly closed container in a cool dark place. The tart hips are a great source of vitamin C as well as A, B, D, and E. Rose hips are also packed with bioflavonoids and possess nearly all of the medicinal proper-

ties of the petals. Rose hip seed oil is a fixed oil (not essential) that is renowned for healing or preventing scar tissue; it regenerates skin, prevents wrinkles, soothes psoriasis and eczema, heals burns, and helps damaged skin regain its natural tone and color.

Medicinal Benefits

» Lifts depression
» Inhibits oxidation
» Relieves muscle spasms
» Boosts libido
» Constricts tissue
» Kills bacteria, viruses, and other pathogens
» Reduces inflammation
» Stimulates digestion
» Loosens phlegm
» Increases bile production

ROSE AND LEMON GULKAND

Rose gulkand is a type of rose jam that originated in the Middle East, where it is used to stimulate digestion. It is cooling and reduces stress. It is also delicious. I started adding lemon, and find it nearly irresistible.

Ingredients

1 quart (1 L) lightly packed highly
 fragrant rose petals

1½ to 2 cups (300 to 400 g) raw sugar

Zest of 1 lemon

⅛ teaspoon ground cardamom

Directions

In a clean quart (1 L) jar, layer 1 inch (2.5 cm) of rose petals. Cover with about ¼ inch (6 mm) of sugar. Repeat. Every few layers, add a bit of the lemon zest and a pinch of the cardamom. Continue until all the ingredients are used, with sugar being the top layer. Cover tightly.

Leave on the windowsill, where the sunlight will break down the petals and the sugar and rose will begin to meld. Every other day, stir the mixture and return it to the windowsill. Continue for a month, and it is done.

This is delicious on scones, ice cream, crepes, and even toast. The delicate flavor of rose with the zip of the lemon and mellowness of the cardamom is unforgettable. This could easily be considered a love spell if that intention is added during the stirring. Feed it to the object of your affections—it just might do the trick.

Yield » 1 quart (1 L)

ROSE MILK BATH

The following recipe can be made with any kind of powdered milk. Goat, cow, and coconut milk are all available in powdered form. Another option is to add 1 cup (235 ml) of fresh milk directly to the bath and brew the rose mixture separately, which would allow the use of soy or nut milks as well, if you prefer. Using powdered milk lets you make it all up ahead and it can even be packaged for gifts, but either way works fine.

Ingredients

2 cups rose petals
 (the most fragrant you can find)
2 cups violet leaves
2 cups (240 g) milk powder
½ cup (40 g) oatmeal

Directions

Combine all the ingredients in an airtight jar. To use, place about ¼ cup of the mixture into a cloth bag and brew it in just boiled water for 10 minutes while the bath runs. Pour the tea (and the bag) into the tub and soak your cares away. Very soothing to dry or windswept skin.

Yield » 12 to 14 applications

ROSE BEADS

There are several old recipes for rose beads that involve cooking the petals for several days in cast iron. This method produces coal black beads. They are lovely, and I've made them a few times, but I am not the patient type. To make rose beads in one day (except the drying), follow this recipe.

Ingredients

1 tablespoon finely powdered rose petals (the deepest color you can find is best)

¼ teaspoon gum tragacanth powder

½ teaspoon red or pink clay

1 tablespoon (15 ml) rose water, or more as needed

Directions

In a bowl, blend the powders and add the rose water. The consistency should resemble modeling clay. Roll the beads with your fingers into the size and shape that you'd like, and string them onto thick wire. I use floral wire from the craft store, the thickest available. Leave about ½ inch (1.3 cm) between beads.

Drape the wires of beads across a box or bowl so that there is circulation beneath the beads. Gently rotate the beads on the wire every 8 or 10 hours. Depending on the size of the beads you make, they might be dry the next day, or it could take several days.

ROSE AND VANILLA ELIXIR

Blessed Maine Herb Farm was awarded first place for this elixir in the Simply Delicious Syrups and Elixirs category at the 2013 International Herb Symposium. Roses uplift the spirit, calm and center the mind, nourish the heart, and encourage love and procreation. They are astringent and tonic to the digestive and eliminative tract. Vanilla beans relax and soothe, warm the gut, bring us into our bodies, offer mild aphrodisiac properties, and taste delicious.

Ingredients

3 to 5 vanilla beans, sliced lengthwise and finely chopped or juiced

1-pint (470 ml) jar loosely filled with fresh rose petals

1 cup (235 ml) high-quality, smooth-tasting brandy

1 cup (320 g) pure raw honey

Directions

Add the vanilla to the jar of roses. Combine the brandy and honey, mix well, and pour over the roses and vanilla. Cover to the rim of the jar and poke with a chopstick to make sure the herbal material is covered. Cap the jar and store in a cool, dark place for 4 to 6 weeks. Strain and decant into a clean bottle.

Take a dropperful of the elixir straight into your mouth, or add to a cup of hot or cold water or tea anytime you need a bit of inspiration, relaxation, or respite. It's an excellent gut-warming digestive aid and is awesome over vanilla ice cream!

Source

Gail Faith Edwards, www.BlessedMaineHerbs.com

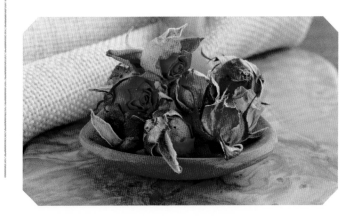

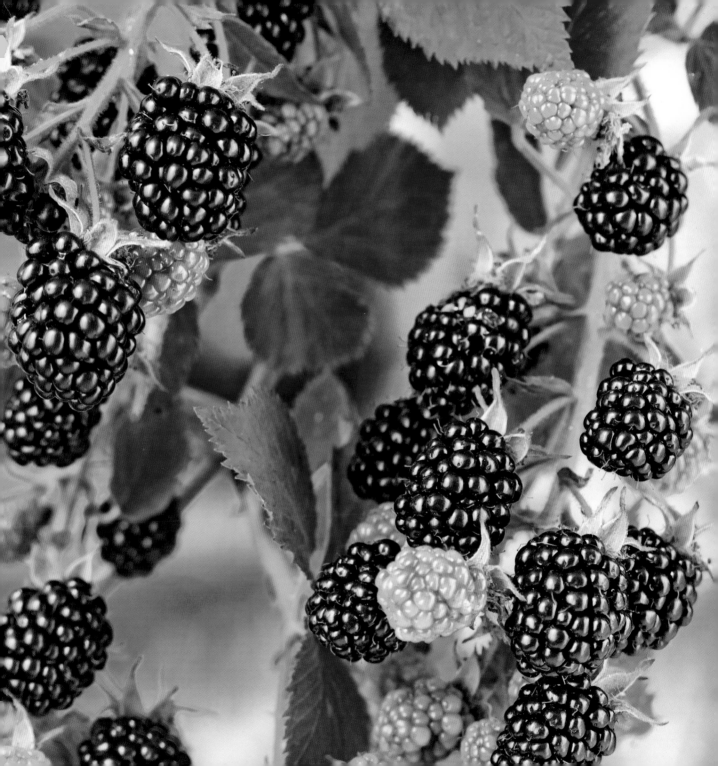

CHAPTER ELEVEN

Raspberry Blackberry

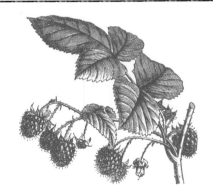

Rubus spp.

Rosaceae family

THERE ARE MANY wild berries that cover the hillsides, fencerows, and woodlands, but the most familiar and easily identified are raspberries and blackberries. Besides being delicious, they have many medicinal properties.

Raspberry time is around midsummer. Blackberries ripen toward the end of the summer.

With a little diligence, you can find wild fruit and other foods almost year-round, depending on the climate. The raspberries that grow wild in my area are "black raspberries" because they are black when ripe (*Rubus occidentalis*). Red raspberry leaf (*Rubus idaeus*) is used medicinally, but the black ones have much of the same properties and plenty of the valuable antioxidants that make so many of the red, blue, and purple berries "superfoods." The pigments in these foods are anthocyanins, a naturally occurring flavonoid, and they have a great deal to offer.

Many in the medical field believe that nearly all disease is caused by inflammation and the steps our body's defense mechanisms take to fight it. Anthocyanins are credited with fighting the free radicals that lead to inflammation. The berries are also antiviral and anticancer, help maintain a healthy blood pressure and prevent heart disease, and may even protect against obesity.

Raspberries and blackberries are aggregate fruits composed of many small, single-seeded drupelets. The drupelets form around the outside of a core, or rasp. When raspberries are picked, the berry slips off the rasp, leaving it behind, and there is an indentation in the fruit where the rasp was. Raspberries are rounded. With blackberries (*Rubus fruticosus*), the receptacle breaks off and remains inside the fruit. When a ripe blackberry is picked, the stem left behind is clean and flat, and the soft white core stays inside the berry. The blackberry is not hollow. If it is not ripe, it will not come away easily from the stem. Blackberries are oblong or even somewhat cylindrical. It came as a great surprise to find that the leaves of these fruits (as well as those of strawberry) make a tea that is delicately flavored like the fruit. Raspberry leaf tea has many wonderful medicinal uses. One of the best known is for toning the uterus and easing childbirth, due to its ability to relax blood vessels and help relax (or contract) smooth muscle. Midwives often recommend it for the last few weeks of pregnancy, and it is possible that a toned, relaxed uterus is more receptive to embryo implantation, making it a good pre-pregnancy choice for those wishing to conceive. Safety of use in the early to late stage of pregnancy is mixed, so I would personally choose to avoid it until a few weeks prior to the due date.

Raspberry leaf tea, as well as the fruits, are cooling in the heat of summer. I enjoy drying the extra fruits and chopping them coarsely to

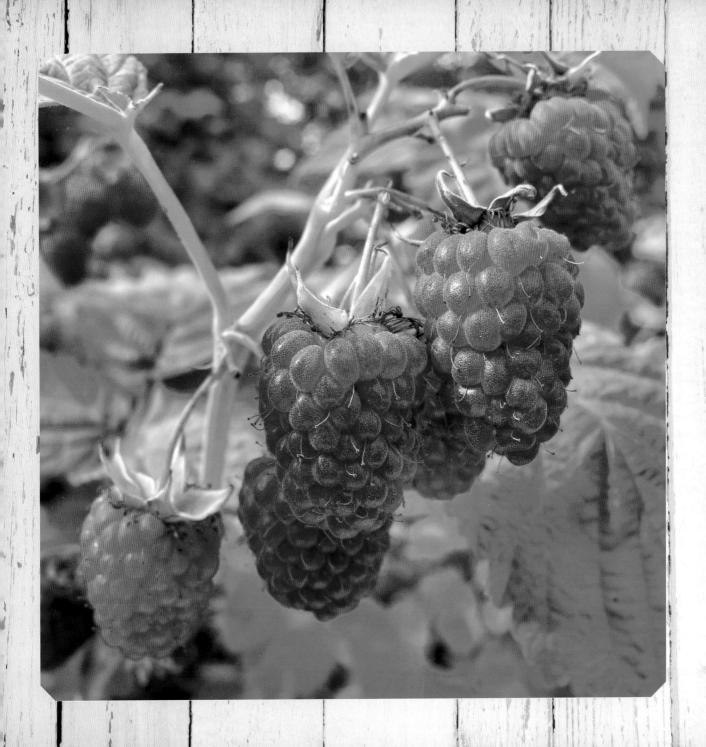

add to tea blends. The berries are loaded with vitamin C and dietary fiber. The leaves have even more to offer, including vitamins A and B complex, iron, calcium, magnesium, phosphorous, and potassium. It can be helpful for leg cramps.

Blackberry has a long history of use, particularly among Native Americans who used root and leaf decoctions for diarrhea. Some used it for hemorrhoids and lung conditions, as well. Ancient Greeks used blackberry for gout, so one of its many nicknames is the goutberry. Another is brambleberry, because of the wild growth habit of the blackberry. The canes can grow over 15 feet (5 m) long in a single season, and the brambles sometimes take over huge areas of several acres.

Blackberry leaf and root bark are both considered to be the medicinal parts of the plant. The leaf and root bark are astringent, diuretic, and rich in tannins. They have long been used in cases of diarrhea and for oral (mucous membrane) inflammation. Hemorrhoids respond to external use of blackberry in the form of a compress or wash.

My grandfather was not much of a drinker, but blackberry brandy was a favorite. I make my own version by filling a jar with fresh, ripe berries, a few leaves, and some root bark, and then covering it completely with brandy for at least several weeks before straining it for use.

Be sure to gather and dry some wild berries and leaves for wild teas full of vitamins and flavor over the winter. The leaves are easy to dry on a screen. Make sure they are completely dry before storing. The berries can be a little tougher, though. I usually put them in a single layer on a cookie sheet lined with baking parchment, and put them in the oven on "warm" for several hours until they have started to dry. They contain a lot of water, so if they aren't dried carefully and quickly, they can mold. The warm oven method has not failed me yet.

Medicinal Benefits

- » Reduces inflammation
- » Kills viruses
- » Prevents cancer
- » Reduces high blood pressure
- » Prevents heart disease
- » Protects against obesity
- » Eases childbirth
- » Eases cramps
- » Treats gout
- » Constricts tissues
- » Promotes urination

BERRY FRUIT LEATHER

We have a beautiful Golden Delicious apple tree, so I always make applesauce first, and then use that as a base for fruit leather. It comes out uniform and sweet, and the applesauce holds the juices from berries that might not have enough substance to make a good leather. You can use store-bought applesauce just as well. Unsweetened is plenty sweet once it dries down.

Ingredients

½ to 1 cup (120 to 235 ml) berry juice (can be one berry or mixed)

2 cups (490 g) applesauce

Directions

Preheat the oven to the lowest setting.

To make the juice, smash the berries with an old-fashioned potato masher or spoon, and heat in a saucepan until the juice runs. Crush well. Strain to obtain all the juice available and remove the seeds. Blend with the applesauce.

Line a large shallow-sided cookie sheet with parchment paper. Some people use plastic wrap, which is tidier, but heated plastic isn't a particularly healthy choice. Spread the blended juice and applesauce to a uniform thickness on the cookie sheet, no more than ¼-inch (6 mm) thick.

Place in the oven for several hours. Check often, and if necessary, rotate the pan. The center of the mixture should be just barely tacky, but not wet when it is finished.

To store, cut into strips, lay on slightly larger strips of waxed paper, and roll up. Keep in a tightly sealed jar. Refrigerate, or eat within a few weeks.

Yield » 12 x 18-inch (30.5 x 45.7 cm) sheet, cut into strips of your choosing

BLACK RASPBERRY PIE

When Mom baked, it was an event. Her baking time was severely restricted, having a panel of phones ringing 24 hours a day and five kids to raise, but occasionally, we found enough black raspberries, and she found enough time to bake them into a pie.

Ingredients

Pastry for an 8-inch (20 cm) two-crust pie
¾ cup (150 g) sugar
¼ cup (30 g) flour
¼ teaspoon ground cinnamon
3 cups (435 g) fresh black raspberries
1 tablespoon (14 g) unsalted butter

Directions

Preheat the oven to 425°F (220°C, or gas mark 7). Line a pie pan with one of the crusts.

In a bowl, combine the sugar, flour, and cinnamon. Add the berries and mix lightly. Pour into the pastry-lined pie pan. Dot with the butter. Cover with the top crust. Seal and flute. Prick the crust with a fork.

Bake until the crust is golden brown and the juices are bubbly and thickened, 35 to 45 minutes.

Yield » 8 servings

GO WITH THE FLOW FOR MEN

This blend promotes healthy prostate function and normalizes urine flow. It combines multiple supportive herbs. This recipe may also be helpful for an enlarged prostate.

Ingredients

2 cups (290 g) red raspberries
Unsalted butter or coconut oil, for greasing
¼ ounce dried ashwagandah
¼ ounce dried saw palmetto
¼ ounce dried powdered turmeric
¼ ounce dried gotu kola
¼ ounce dried nettle
¼ ounce dried raspberry leaf
2 cups (400 g) organic sugar or (640 g) honey

Directions

Make a juice from the berries. In a pot, cover the raspberries with water plus 1 inch (2.5 cm), and boil until the berries have popped. Strain. Set aside 1 cup (235 ml).

Grease a mold with butter or coconut oil. If you don't have a mold, you will roll the candy later.

In a small stainless steel pot, boil the ashwagandah, saw palmetto, and turmeric in water to cover for 25 minutes. If the liquid gets low, add more water in ¼ cup (60 ml) increments. Turn off the heat and add the guto kola, nettle and raspberry leaf. Let sit, covered, for 25 minutes. Cool and strain the mixture using cheesecloth. Reserve ½ cup (120 ml) of the tea and compost the herbs.

In a pot, combine the sugar, reserved berry liquid, and reserved tea; bring to a boil. Cook the mixture, stirring constantly, until the syrup reaches 290° to 300°F (143° to 150°C) on a candy thermometer (this will take a while). Place a drop or two of the syrup into a bowl full of ice water. If the syrup turns and stays hard (crack stage), then you know it's ready. If it is still soft and sticky, it needs to keep cooking.

Pour the syrup into the molds. You can remove the drops from the mold once they have cooled. If you don't have a mold, when the syrup has cooled and is pliable, begin pulling off small pieces and rolling between the palms of your greased hands, forming a small ball. Work quickly because the mixture hardens pretty fast.

Store in a cool, dry place.

Yield »
The yield is dependent on the size of your drops. I make some larger for adults and some smaller for children.

Source
Marita Orr, www.withseedsofintention.com

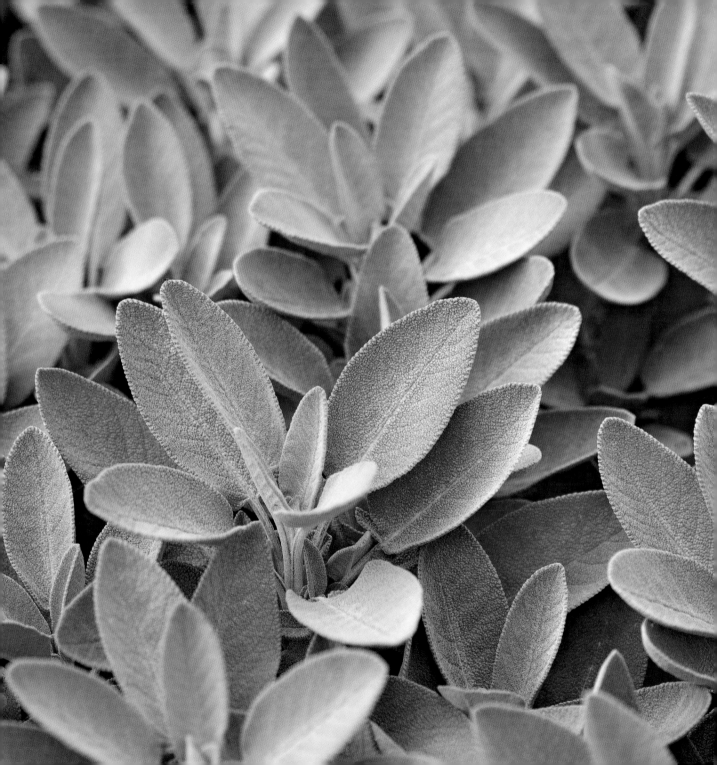

CHAPTER TWELVE

Sage

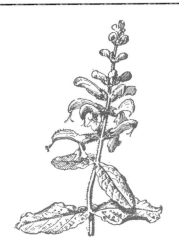

Salvia spp.

Labiatae family

THERE ARE QUITE A FEW cultivars and species of salvia. Most of the time when we talk about sage, we're describing garden sage, but the white ceremonial sage from the desert Southwest, the striking pineapple sage that draws hummingbirds, the tall, abundantly flowering Mexican bush sage, the enormous, showy clary sage, and all the varieties in between also have their own uses. Some sages are mainly ornamental, some are grown for their scent, many are amazing medicine, and some make splendid tea. We do not think of this culinary herb nearly as often as we should in cooking. It has a lot to offer.

Sage leaves are strong and thick with a surface that appears pebbled. They remind me somewhat of an exaggerated tongue. Because it is astringent, it helps shrink inflamed mucous membranes of the mouth and throat.

Sage contains a wide range of valuable and healing volatile oils, flavonoids (including apigenin, diosmetin, and luteolin), and phenolic acids, including rosmarinic acid, found in the herb rosemary. This acid is readily available for absorption in the gastrointestinal tract and from there can reduce the number of inflammatory messaging molecules, thereby helping to reduce inflammation. Additionally, sage contains antioxidant enzymes that combine with the flavonoids and acids, giving it a special ability to stabilize damage to cells from free radicals. Due to this unique combination, sage is a powerful herb for people with conditions caused by or worsened by inflammation, such as rheumatoid arthritis, asthma, and atherosclerosis.

The name Salvia derives from the Latin *salvere*, meaning "to be saved" or "salvation." There are many herbs that lead me down the road of wondering which came first, the herb or the word. Sage is one such herb. When we use the word *sage* in a non-herbal context, it refers to one who holds much wisdom. We look for "sage advice." So it is interesting indeed that eating sage enhances memory due to the flavonoids and most likely rosmarinic acid. Sage is an amazing source of several B-complex vitamins, including folic acid, thiamin, pyridoxine, and riboflavin. Plenty of vitamins C and A, plus minerals like potassium, zinc, calcium, iron, manganese, copper, and magnesium, make this a valuable food way beyond what it can do for a turkey a couple of times a year!

Garden sage (*Salvia officinalis*) and the many varieties of Salvia are used anytime there is an abundance of moisture. Mothers wishing to dry up milk production have relied on sage for centuries. Menopausal hot flashes sometimes respond to sage tea or tincture. Colds where there is a lot of mucus can benefit from sage. Sage is also calming and grounding both internally and externally. It has traditionally been used to treat fevers and promote sleep.

Clary sage, *Salvia sclarea*

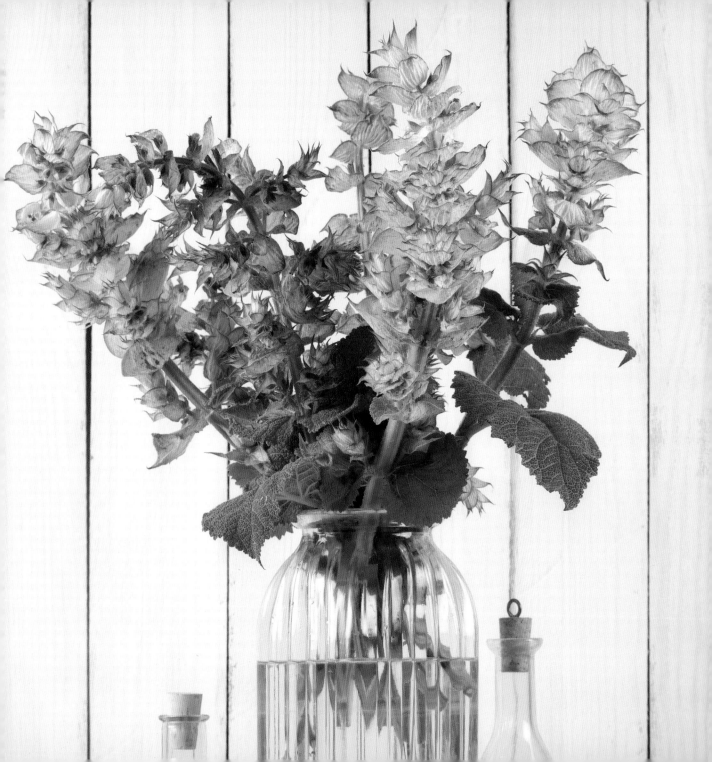

The herb is found to be capable of killing *E. coli* and is a strong antifungal. Making use of powdered sage in products such as homemade toothpaste, liniments, or vinegars can solve many problems due to dampness, sweat, and fungus. An infused vinegar is terrific on oily skin or as a hair rinse for oily hair, and sage vinegar can dry up an oozing poison ivy or oak rash in no time flat.

Clary sage (*Salvia sclarea*) in particular is considered a woman's herb in part because of its estrogen-stimulating action. The essential oil was first described to me by a friend, describing how after the death of her mother, she felt that a few drops of clary sage essential oil in the bathtub each night was the only thing that got her through. Naturally, I assumed that this would be a heady, floral scent with a grounding semi-sharp sage fragrance. My first sniff of clary was quite a shock, and it took me a while to develop a fondness for it, but now I "get" it. Clary sage essential oil's scent is thick, deep, and earthy. I can imagine that it might give one the sense of crawling into a safe, mossy cave. The plant itself is large with immense leaves that bear little resemblance to the regular garden sages. The flower spikes are nearly 12 inches (30.5 cm) of glorious pinkish purple blooms. In addition to garden sage's properties of being antiseptic, antispasmodic, astringent, and antibacterial, clary sage is antidepressant, making it a fitting herb for PMS and various women's issues.

Some of the more ornamental salvias are fun to grow and make delicious teas, but don't seem to have the same medicinal qualities or the rugged perennial growth of garden sage.

Sage's deep, rich, earthy quality is unmatched for culinary uses. Try placing a sage leaf around a shrimp before wrapping it in bacon and baking. Pork and sage was, at one time, as famous as sage stuffing for Thanksgiving dinner. Sage has the ability to aid in the digestion of fat, so it was included in fatty meat recipes.

Medicinal Benefits

» Reduces inflammation
» Inhibits oxidation
» Enhances memory
» Kills fungi
» Treats oily skin and hair

SAGE TEA

This tea is perfect for a sore, scratchy throat or when a bug is getting you down. I really like to use a licorice root stick as a stirrer for the added soothing properties.

Ingredients

2 teaspoons dried sage or 5 or 6 fresh leaves
1 cup (235 ml) boiling water
Juice of ½ lemon
Honey to taste

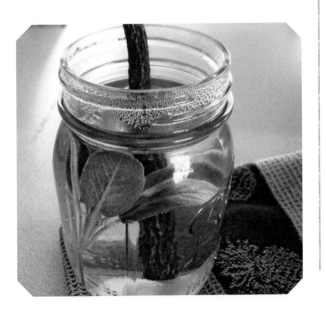

Directions

Steep the sage in the boiling water for at least 5 minutes. Remove the sage, add the lemon juice and honey, and drink.

Note: You can make sage and lemon honey ahead, and just add that to hot water. Just like making a vinegar or a tincture, chop the sage fine, slice the lemon thin, and when you've filled the jar two-thirds full with them, pour a good-quality local honey (raw is best) over them, using a chopstick to make sure everything is well coated. I keep that in the refrigerator until it is needed. The honey is a great preservative.

Yield » 1 cup (235 ml)

HIKER'S RASH RELIEF

I use this all summer long on rashes from plants, bug bites, and all of summer's skin itchies. It is inexpensive and easy to make. You can skip an herb or two if you can't find it, but don't skip the sage! Use about equal parts herbs, with a heavy hand on the sage.

Ingredients

Sage leaves (I use 'Berggarten' for its very high ratio of essential oil)

Plantain leaves

Yarrow flowers and leaves

Jewelweed (cut early in the summer when the stems are succulent and juicy)

Apple cider vinegar

Directions

Combine the herbs in a jar and add apple cider vinegar to cover; allow to steep for a month if possible. Strain enough to fill a spray bottle and use. I leave the rest soaking for as long as I can.

Yield » As desired

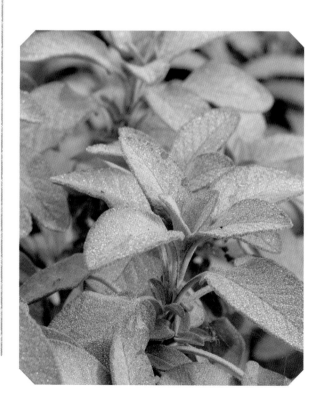

FRIED SAGE LEAVES

I resisted these for years, thinking they didn't sound very good. What a huge mistake that was! Just last year I decided to give it a go to use as a garnish on some butternut squash soup, and it wasn't easy to restrain myself from eating them all before the soup was even ready.

Ingredients

2 tablespoons (28 g) unsalted butter
Whole sage leaves

Directions

Melt the butter in a frying pan and then slip the whole sage leaves in, heating until they get crisp, like buttery, savory little chips of flavor . . . where was I? Oh right. Drain on a paper towel. These will keep at room temperature for a couple of days if they are in an airtight container.

Yield » As desired

SALVIA FRITTA

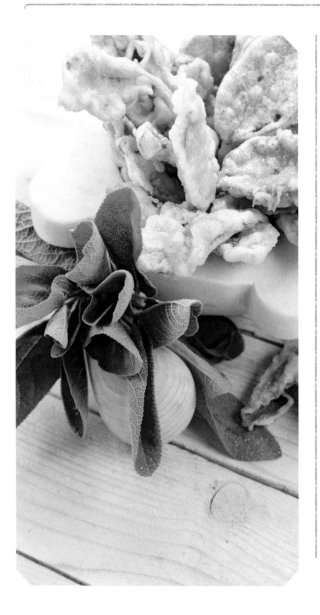

This is a bit more complicated method of making fried sage leaves.

Ingredients

1 cup (226 g) coconut oil
¼ cup (40 g) flour
¼ cup (30 g) cornstarch
½ cup (120 ml) soda water
16 to 24 perfect sage leaves
Sea salt

Directions

Heat the oil in a frying pan. While it heats, combine the flour, cornstarch, and soda water in a bowl and whisk well. Dredge the sage leaves in the batter. When the oil is good and hot, add 4 or 5 of the leaves to the pan, and fry until golden brown. Drain on paper towels. Repeat until all the leaves are fried. I'm not sure how long these will keep. It's never happened.

Save the oil, which will be infused with sage flavor. You can use it to cook poultry, potatoes, or veggies later.

Yield » 16 to 24 sage leaves

SAGE PESTO

This recipe uses garlic scapes, the hollow blades that grow in the spring just prior to a bloom. The scapes must be cut to prevent that bloom, keeping the energy of the plant focused on the bulb of garlic under the ground. Scapes have become a bit of a delicacy in recent years, and are often found at farmers' markets in the spring.

Ingredients

⅔ cup (160 g) olive oil, or more as needed, divided

1 cup chopped garlic scapes

1 cup fresh sage

¼ cup (50 g) chopped walnuts, toasted

¼ cup (35 g) grated Parmesan cheese

Directions

In blender, combine ¼ cup (80 ml) of the olive oil, the garlic scapes, and the sage. Blend on high. While the ingredients are blending, add the remaining ¼ cup (80 ml) olive oil in a stream. If the mixture is dry, add more oil. Add the nuts and blend briefly. Mix in the Parmesan cheese by hand.

Yield » 3 cups (720 g)

Source   Betty Pillsbury, www.GreenSpiralHerbs.com

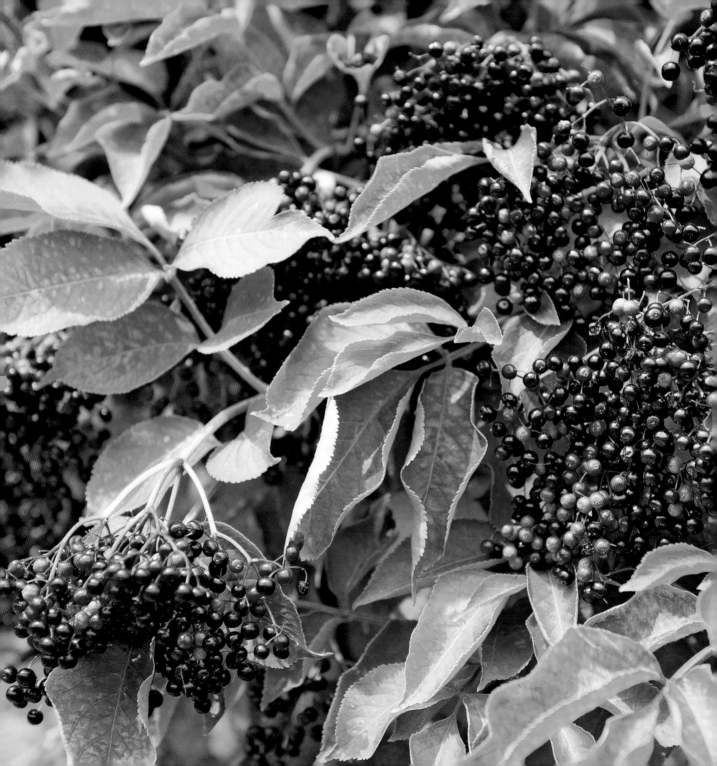

CHAPTER THIRTEEN

Elder

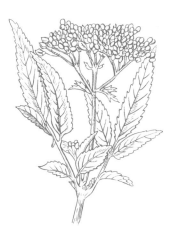

Sambucus spp.

Adoxaceae family

ELDER BUSHES seem to pop up everywhere in fields, meadows, and suburban yards. This generous plant is spread by birds and animals eating the berries and dispersing the seeds. Unassuming, delicate, frothy flower heads in spring and early summer are followed by jewel-like garnet to black berries. A delicate floral scent wafts on the breeze. Elder was preceded only by chamomile when I first set about to find useful wild plants, so elder and I go way back. It would be unthinkable now to face winter without a good supply of elder's bounty.

Elder has been an amazing ally to humanity from before recorded time, but there is vast and conflicting lore associated with the plant. Depending on who does the telling, the elder plant is considered either protective or dangerous. For instance, elder can protect one from witches or the wood can become a magic wand. Various sources explain that the wood repels lightning, while others say that it draws lightning. Nearly all ancient writings consider the plant to be female and suggest that you ask the old lady within for permission before harvesting. Branches of elder wood have long been used for flutes and similar musical instruments because the outer bark encircles a soft pithy center that is easily hollowed.

Elderberries and elderflowers have been used medicinally for colds and flu for many generations. Some early recorded instances of the berries date to ancient Greece. Some herbalists prefer to use the flowers, while others swear by the berries, but either way, this plant offers us great benefits. In the eastern United States, the *S. Canadensis* variety is the wild bush found in meadows and woodlands, while on the West Coast, the wild berries are coated with a pale blue powdery blush. That variety is *S. cerulean* (sometimes also known as *S. Mexicana*). There are many cultivars. All of the purple-black berried varieties are considered to have similar properties. Around the world, there are various traditional dishes and beverages based on both the elderflower and the elderberry. Elderberries can be found in parts of Europe, Asia, South America, and most of the Northern Hemisphere, with many varieties being represented, depending on the location.

In the spring, the flowers appear on large flat umbels up to 15 inches (38 cm) in diameter. The flowers are gathered when they are full and pale cream colored. If left to develop fruit, the berries appear in early fall ready to be harvested when they are dark and nearly black in color. High in vitamin C, the flowers steeped into a tea are anti-inflammatory, antiviral, and anticatarrhal, and induce perspiration, helping to hurry a virus on its way. They work as a potassium-sparing diuretic, clearing tissues and mucous membranes of excess fluid.

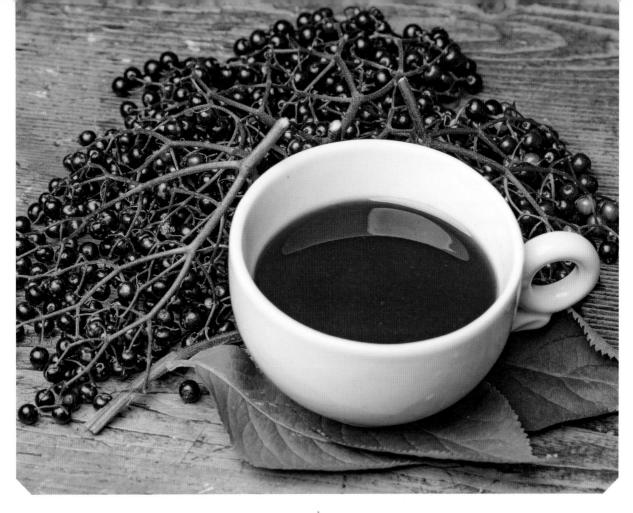

In addition to internal use, elderflowers love the skin. A strong elderflower water infusion on a compress is said to lighten freckles, age spots, and darkish patches of skin. Historically, it was also applied liberally to lift the heat of sunburn, rosacea, boils, and carbuncles. Soothing and healing to the skin, elderflower is used in lotions, facials, and facial steams and spa treatments.

Elderberries are crammed with good stuff! There are many bioflavonoids, including extremely powerful antioxidant anthocyanins that create an inhospitable environment for the replication of viruses. When a virus is unable to replicate, it quickly washes from the body. Flavonoids (the blue and purple pigments) have antibacterial, antiviral, antitumor, anti-inflammatory, antiallergenic, and vasodilatory effects on the body. Many people find relief within hours of taking an elderberry preparation for flu symptoms. If taken every few hours for a few days, it can completely wipe out a stubborn virus. Research has been conducted on elderberry's effect on flu with great results, and many state agencies now encourage the propagation of elderberry as a crop. Centuries of empirical evidence have also shown this to be true, but a little controlled research never hurts. The commercial preparation Sambucol has long been used for decades by the Israeli Air Force when it is necessary to quickly recover from cold or flu.

The medicinal components have been found to be heat-resistant, and thus able to be cooked, making them easy to incorporate into a daily "food as medicine" regimen during the winter months. The seeds contain small amounts of a glycoside, which metabolizes into cyanide (as do many fruit seeds), and cooking the berries helps activate the medicinal properties and releases the undesirable cyanide residue. Eating more than a small handful of raw berries may cause gastric upset in some people.

It is very easy to grow elderberry. Branches lie across the ground and root, or they can even be rooted in water. The shrubby bushes will grow in partial shade, but are even happier in full sun. They like lots of water, but will flourish in drier settings if there's plenty of rain. Once

established, they will withstand a lot of neglect, being a weed after all.

There are a few pests that will cut into the harvest. Tent caterpillars must be watched for and removed at first sighting. Birds love the berries, and if there isn't enough other wild food available, they'll eat them all. Fruit flies can also attack the berries, but an organic pesticide containing Spinosad and vinegar traps may take care of the problem.

There are so many ways to use the flowers and berries. My favorite preparation is to simply freeze the berries in 1-quart (1 L) bags so that they are ready for anything during the winter. Both the berries and the flowers are easily dried for later use.

Medicinal Benefits

- » Treats cold and flu
- » Promotes urination
- » Soothes and heals skin
- » Kills viruses
- » Promotes sweating
- » Reduces inflammation of the airways

ELDERBERRY JUICE

The juice can be frozen or canned. Freeze it in 1-cup (235 ml) portions in a flat container, large enough that the frozen juice is less than ½-inch (1.3 cm) thick. It is so easy to just break off a piece when needed.

Ingredients

1 quart fresh elderberries or 1 cup (150 g) dried

1 quart (940 ml) water (if using dried berries), plus water to cover

Directions

Place the fresh rinsed berries into a pan and add just enough water to avoid scorching. Heat to a simmer and muddle to help release the juice as the heat starts to pop the berries. A potato masher is great for this purpose. Continue gently heating and occasionally mashing until most of the berries have burst and turned to juice. Pour through a fine-mesh strainer to capture the seeds, or line a strainer with a piece of cheese-cloth.

This is a fairly concentrated juice, and 1 cup (235 ml) taken in 1-tablespoon (15 ml) portions four times a day for three days is enough to get a person through a viral threat.

If using dried berries, soak the berries in 4 cups (940 ml) water overnight and proceed as above.

Yield » 3 cups (705 ml)

ELDERBERRY EXTRACT/TINCTURE

This is one of the few tinctures that you can make quarts (liters) of each year, and you'll probably either use it yourself or share it with family and friends. Once you see how quickly it can stop a virus in its tracks, you'll be sharing with everyone you know.

Ingredients

Dried or fresh elderberries
Menstruum (vodka or alcohol of choice) to cover

Directions

If using dried material, fill a 1-pint (470 ml) jar one-third full before adding liquid (menstruum is the technical term for the solvent or carrier used in an extract, tincture, or elixir). If using fresh herbs, fill loosely to the top. Follow the instructions on page 12.

Yield » 1 pint (470 ml)

ELDERBERRY SYRUP

This syrup is so delicious it can be used to sweeten tea or spread on toast and pancakes, and the kids just might tell you the second they feel the tiniest bit scratchy in the throat.

Ingredients

1 cup (150 g) dried elderberries or 3 cups (450 g) fresh or frozen

Zest and juice from 1 lemon

2- to 3-inch (5 to 7.5 cm) piece of ginger root, grated

6-inch (15 cm) piece of cinnamon bark, broken

5 cardamom pods

1 vanilla bean or 1 teaspoon vanilla extract

3 cups (705 ml) water if using dried berries or 1 cup (235 ml) if using fresh or frozen

1½ cups (160 g) honey

Yield » 3 cups (705 ml)

Directions

Put all the ingredients except the honey into a saucepan and bring to a boil over medium heat. Lower the heat, and slowly simmer for 30 minutes. Allow to cool, and then strain, squeezing all the good liquid from the solids. Measure, and return the infusion to a simmer until there is 1½ cups (355 ml) liquid. Allow to cool slightly and stir in the honey until it is well incorporated.

Sugar can be used instead of honey. To do that, measure the liquid after cooking, and add twice as much sugar as there is liquid. For example, if there is 1 cup (235 ml) of liquid, use 2 cups (400 g) of sugar. Stir to dissolve the sugar and then bring to a boil for 3 to 5 minutes to reduce slightly. The amount of sugar or honey is necessary as a preservative, so if you choose to use less, it must be refrigerated and used within a month or two.

Most of the spices in the recipe can be treated as optional (except ginger, I love that warming ginger in there), and I initially started adding them to the recipe for the flavor. It was a pleasant surprise to learn years later that cardamom, a seed that is often used in Indian dishes, has antiviral properties, too!

Refrigerate for longer storage.

ELDER TEA BLEND

This is a great blend for kicking that bug before it gets a foothold.

Ingredients

1 tablespoon dried elderberries

1 tablespoon dried elderflowers

1 tablespoon minced crystallized ginger

1 tablespoon dried peppermint (substitute half or all with holy basil if available)

Directions

Combine the herbs in a jar and mix well. Use a rounded teaspoonful of the blend per 1 cup (235 ml) of boiling water and steep for at least 5 minutes. Add honey and a lemon slice, pull on warm socks, and relax.

Yield » ¼ cup, enough for 10 to 12 cups of tea

ELDERBERRY PIE

This is a delicious, juicy berry pie for anytime, but if there's a virus going around, it's just one more way to get a dose of elderberry prevention.

Ingredients

Pastry for a 9-inch (23 cm) two-crust pie
3 cups (450 g) elderberries
¼ teaspoon salt
1⅛ cups (225 g) sugar
3¾ tablespoons (56 ml) lemon juice
2¼ tablespoons 18 g) cornstarch
2 tablespoons (28 g) unsalted butter

Directions

Preheat the oven to 425°F (220°C, or gas mark 7). Line a 9-inch (23 cm) pie pan with one of the crusts.

Combine the elderberries, salt, sugar, lemon juice and cornstarch in a saucepan over medium heat and cook until thick. Pour into the pastry-lined pie pan. Dot with the butter. Cover with the top crust. Seal and flute. Prick the crust with a fork.

Bake for 10 minutes, then lower the oven temperature to 350°F (180°C, or gas mark 4) and bake for 30 more minutes, or until the crust is golden brown and the juices are bubbly and thickened.

Yield » 8 servings

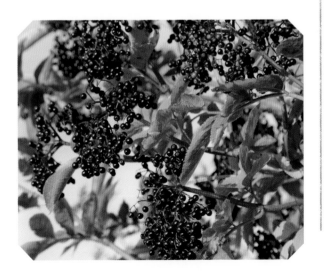

ELDERBERRY APPLE FRUIT LEATHER

I make fresh apple and pear sauce from the trees here on the farm. Commercial applesauce works well too, but if it has a lot of liquid, strain it out prior to use.

Ingredients

1 cup (235 ml) elderberry juice
2 cups (490 g) apple or pear sauce

Directions

Preheat the oven to its lowest setting. Line a 12 x 18-inch (30.5 x 45.7 cm) rimmed baking sheet with parchment paper.

Combine the juice and applesauce and stir to blend well. Spread the mixture thinly and evenly on the prepared baking sheet. Place in the oven and leave it for several hours, until it is just barely tacky to the touch and peels away from the parchment easily. You can do this in the evening and leave it overnight if you wish.

Cut the leather into strips and wind it around waxed paper to store for later use. Refrigerate or freeze unless it is to be used within a few days. You can freeze it so that it is ready for use in winter.

Yield » 12 x 18-inch (30.5 x 45.7 cm) sheet, cut into strips of your choice

ELDERBERRY LIQUEUR

Liqueurs are descendants of herbal medicines, made as early as the thirteenth century. Early medicinal lore has them romantically brewed by Italian monks in the idyllic pastoral countryside. You can make liqueurs with vodka, but I like to use brandy, which is distilled wine, aged in casks. It's not as harsh as grain alcohol or vodka, and when warmed has a marvelous aromatic fragrance. Elderberry wine is known as a tonic to be taken regularly to boost immunity. Elderberry liqueur can be sipped as an enjoyable nightcap for tonic purposes, and warmed it takes on an additional role, opening bronchial and sinus passages, providing soothing comfort for a sore throat, and relieving chest congestion.

Ingredients

2 cups fresh elderberries or 1 cup dried

1 quart (1 L) brandy (if using dried, add 1 cup [235 ml] for soaking)

3 or 4 strips of citrus rind (pith removed)

1 cup (360 g) honey, or to taste

Directions

If using dried elderberries, place in a bowl, cover with brandy, and soak overnight. Add the berries (do not strain off the soaking brandy), brandy, and citrus (lemon is my favorite) rind to a slow cooker. Cover. Using a candy thermometer, keep the mixture at 145° to 150°F (63° to 65.5°C) for 3 to 5 hours. Be very careful not to overheat. If your slow cooker runs at a higher temperature on low, shorten the infusion time. Cool, strain, and gently press through a muslin cloth. Add honey to taste.

Stir well and pour into a sterilized container. Store in a cool, dark place or refrigerate.

Yield » 1 quart (1 L)

Option

Your imagination and personal taste are the only limits for additives. Some of my favorites to add to the infusion stage are cinnamon sticks, whole cloves, coarsely chopped nutmeg, turmeric, cardamom, hawthorn berries, juniper berries, raspberries, hibiscus flowers, feverfew, lavender, rosemary, sage, fennel seed, melissa, and thyme.

Source
Marcia Elston, www.wingedseed.com

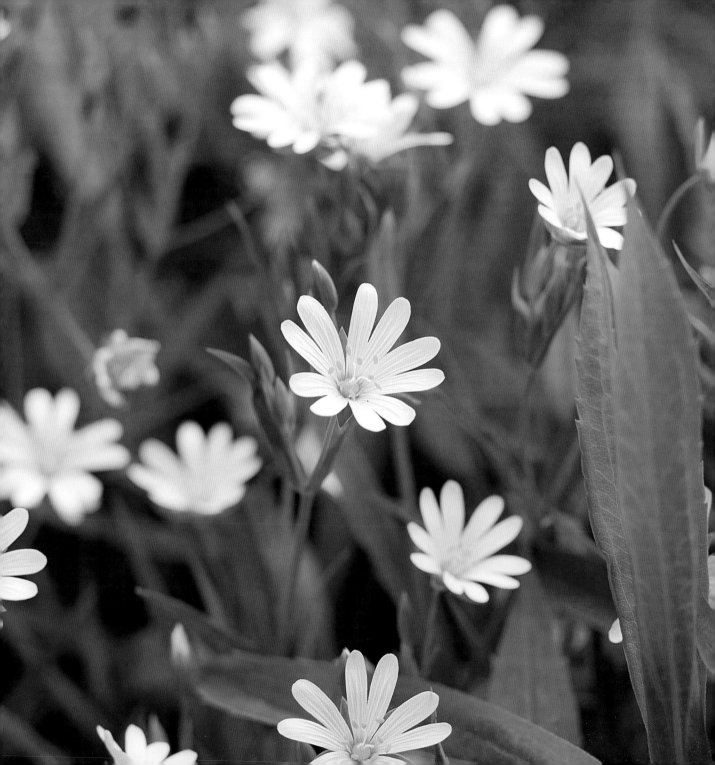

CHAPTER FOURTEEN

Chickweed

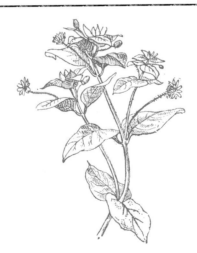

Stellaria media

Caryophyllaceae family

CHICKWEED (*Stellaria media*) is one of the first herbs that many backyard herbalists learn about, and for good reason; it is widely available. Not only does chickweed grow prolifically in temperate climates, but it can also be found growing under snow in the middle of winter. It is one of the first spring greens to wave its pretty little head, and although it gets leggy and dies way back in the heat of summer, there is another full wave in autumn that persists many times through the winter. It is a cool-weather annual, native to Europe. Here on our evergreen farm, the chickweed is nestled under the boughs of the trees nearly year-round. It loves shady, damp areas with rich soil, but can be found in early summer or fall in full sun.

Perhaps because this plant is so ubiquitous, it is also one that I am most often asked to identify. Even herbalists who have been working with plants for years want help with a solid identification. Chickweed is one of the many small, earth-hugging plants that form mats along the ground. When weeding the garden, it can be rewarding to pull up chickweed because while it spreads out over a large area, there is only a small (but deceptively strong and deep) thready root. Covering such a large bit of real estate often means that there aren't other weeds to pull, but chickweed is quick to throw down seeds, too.

The smooth, emerald green leaves are typically about the size of a pinky fingernail, although in the lushness of spring before they bloom, I've seen them up to 1 inch (2.5 cm) long and nearly as wide. They grow in sets, across from each other on the stem, and they almost hug the stem at the base of each leaf, not having leaf stems. There are spaces along the stem of about 1½ inches (3.8 cm) between leaf sets. Shooting out from where the leaves hug the stem are tiny stems that hold the flowers. These flower stems are almost as thin as horsehair. The flowers are white, about ¼ inch (6 mm) across, and each appears to have ten petals. There are really only five petals, with each petal deeply divided. The sepals are longer than the petals. The stem is round, mostly green with a purplish blush. When you crush it, you can feel the crunchiness of it, but it isn't hollow. The stems have a single vertical row of hairs that switches back and forth between leaf sets. After reaching a height of about 3 inches (7.5 cm), the stems, which have a bit of elasticity to them, grow along the ground, and can be several feet long.

Cerastium vulgatum (mouse-ear chickweed) is a lookalike sometimes confused with chickweed, but it is a much darker green, more compact, and coarser. Stellaria leaves are thin and nearly translucent, while Cerastium leaves are stout and sturdy.

Chickweed is packed with iron, calcium, magnesium, manganese, silicon, zinc, phosphorus, potassium, copper, carotenes, and vitamins B and C. Many herbalists swear by chickweed for weight loss because of the saponins that break up fat cells while balancing metabolism. Imagine how welcome those greens must have been in the very early spring after months of heavy salted meats and root vegetables! It has long been used alone and in combination with other herbs as a spring tonic.

Chickweed cools inflammation both inside and out with its demulcent qualities. You can make a simple poultice by placing crushed chickweed directly on the skin, or it can be chopped, heated to release moisture, and wrapped in cheesecloth or something similar to rest on the skin. This can be very soothing and useful for dry or itchy rashes, eczema, psoriasis, poison ivy, or blisters from herpes or shingles.

Another one of chickweed's remarkable qualities is its ability to draw impurities from the skin, making it perfect for things like boils, infections, bee stings, insect bites, or splinters. The plant is so common and accessible that I must confess I sometimes forget all about it. Such was the case a few years ago when, pulling out old bamboo poles from winter storage to stake some tomatoes, I managed to drive a splinter directly into the pad of my thumb. I soaked it in hot water full of Epsom salts, tried duct tape, dug around with a needle and tweezers, and could not get to it. Finally,

I turned to my herbalist friends and asked for advice. Chickweed! It required two poultices of chopped, crushed chickweed about an hour or two apart, and out poked the end of the splinter. Just like that.

With chickweed being such a wonderful medicinal food plant, shouldn't we be getting it onto our plates and into our teacups? In very large amounts, it can have a mild laxative effect, so that would be a sign to back down from it. Chickweed can be so easily incorporated into many dishes. I was happily stunned to find it as part of a greens garnish on my plate at an upscale restaurant last year. Chickweed can be added to eggs, soups, pasta, rice, or potato dishes, eaten as a vegetable all by itself, or hidden in with grains or meatloaf. It's got a lot more to offer than you might realize. And let's face it—the price is right!

Medicinal Benefits

- » Promotes weight loss
- » Lubricates joints
- » Soothes and heals skin
- » Reduces inflammation
- » Draws out impurities

CHICKWEED TINCTURE

It is best to use a high alcohol content in order to get chickweed's constituents into the mix. If you have access to grain alcohol, chickweed responds well to it.

Ingredients

2 cups chickweed
Alcohol to cover

Directions

Coarsely chop by hand or with a food processor enough chickweed to loosely fill a pint (470 ml) canning jar. Cover with alcohol. Allow to steep for 3 to 6 weeks, shaking the bottle occasionally. The chickweed will be colorless when the tincture is ready. Take chickweed tincture by the dropperful up to several times a day. It can be mixed with tea or juice if you prefer.

CHICKWEED VINEGAR

Chickweed is full of great minerals, and vinegar is one of the best ways to make them available in a stable, storable way. It's great for salad dressings and is not a bad way to take some medicine when mixed with juice. Make it just like the tincture above, but instead of alcohol, use a good-quality vinegar.

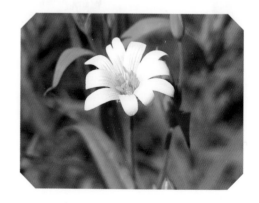

CHICKWEED AND PLANTAIN BALM

This is a classic combination for pulling out infection or toxins, while soothing and encouraging healing.

Ingredients

2 cups coarsely chopped chickweed
2 cups coarsely chopped plantain
1 cup (235 ml) olive oil
2 tablespoons (28 g) beeswax

Directions

Place the chickweed, plantain, and oil in a pan, stirring to get it well combined, and heat to a slow, not-quite-simmer for about 15 minutes. Remove from the heat, cover, and let steep for a few hours or overnight. Strain well.

To make the salve, combine the oil and beeswax in a saucepan. Heat until the wax is melted. When the mixture cools down but is still liquid, pour into wide-mouth jar(s).

Yield » 1 cup (235 ml)

REFRESHING CHICKWEED WATER

This is reputed to be a "flush" and helpful for weight loss, too.

Ingredients

1 quart (1 L) water

2 cups (470 ml) chickweed tea, moderately strong (or 1 tablespoon [15 ml] chickweed tincture)

1 lemon, thinly sliced

1 cucumber, sliced

6 to 8 mint leaves

Directions

Combine all the ingredients in a large pitcher. Drink throughout the day.

Yield » 6 cups (1410 ml)

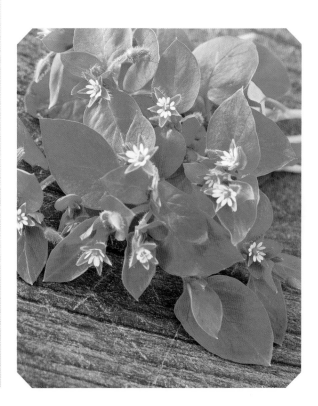

SPRING TONIC OXYMEL

Chickweed is one of the blessings of springtime, and I make the most of it with this oxymel. Oxymels are a mixture of honey and vinegar used medicinally and as the menstruum (solvent for extracting) for plant medicines just like tinctures. It's really old-school herbalism that has its roots all the way back to ancient Greek medicine.

Ingredients

2 tablespoons chickweed
1 tablespoon dandelion leaf
1 tablespoon nettle leaf
1 tablespoon red clover blossom
½ cup (180 g) honey
½ cup (120 ml) apple cider vinegar

Directions

If using dried herbs, fill a 1-pint (470 ml) jar one-fourth to one-third with the plant material (if fresh, then fill the jar half to two-thirds). Combine the honey and vinegar in a saucepan, and warm until you can stir the honey into the vinegar. Pour into the jar until full and stir well to remove air bubbles. Place waxed paper over the top and screw the lid on—the waxed paper will help protect the metal from the vinegar. Shake it gently every day for 3 to 4 weeks, and then pour into a mesh strainer lined with cheesecloth. Gather up the cheesecloth and press to extract as much from the plant material as possible.

This makes a great nutritional tonic for when you need the extra boost—when you're sick, stressed, or simply too busy to eat right. It's like a yummy multivitamin. I take it regularly in the winter when I'm feeling the need for a touch of spring and summer magic during the long, dark, cold days. You can take it by the tablespoonful straight up. I find it is wonderful as a salad dressing or tossed over some freshly steamed veggies with a touch of sea salt, combining the worlds of food and medicine.

Yield » 6 ounces (180 ml)

Source   Michael Blackmore, Mad Crow Herbalism, www.madcrowherbals.com

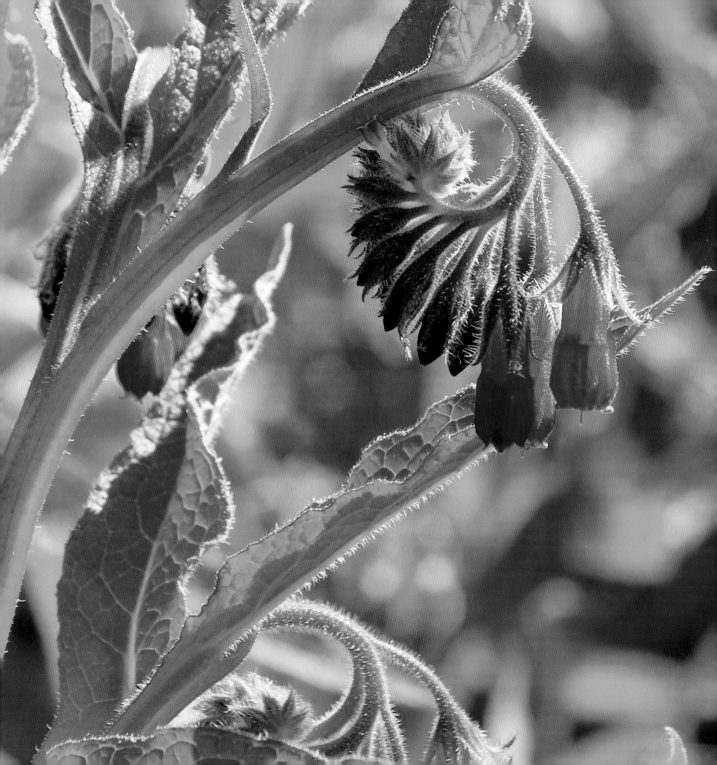

CHAPTER FIFTEEN

Comfrey

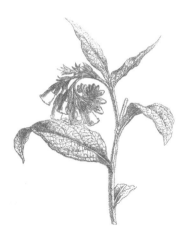

Symphytum officinale

Boraginaceae family

SUCH A GENEROUS healing herb, comfrey, of the Borage family, *Boraginaceae*, grows so abundantly that it can take over entire fields if left to its own devices. In early summer magnificent deep green leaves frame the purple blooms as they unfurl toward the sky.

In the home garden, it helps to keep it in partial shade and to monitor the roots and seeds closely. Bits of root left behind will sprout new plants. Comfrey is worth any trouble it might cause, though. Bruises, strains, and injuries such as *plantar fasciitis* respond beautifully to poultices and compresses of comfrey. It contains *allantoin*, the active ingredient in commercially made salves like Neosporin. Due to its mucilaginous action, wounds are soothed and remain suppler, facilitating healing. In fact, it heals wounds so well and so quickly that you must clean a wound prior to its use, lest infectious matter remain inside while the wound heals around it, causing an abscess.

A soothing bath with a comfrey infusion is superb after a long day in the garden. It can even help with sunburn. The name *Symphytum* comes from the Greek and is a combination of words that mean "grow together" and "plant." Indeed, nicknames such as knitbone, bruisewort, and slippery root help clarify uses its as medicine. Often plants are named for their appearance or growth habit, but in this case it describes the action of the plant's medicine.

When my sister and I had an herb shop, we carried a comfrey and goldenseal salve. A woman limped in one day and lifted her pant leg to show us a very sore, very deep ulcer on her ankle. It was two or three fingers' width in diameter, and at least one finger width deep. Nothing was helping. She decided to try a little jar of salve, and came back a week later for more, once again showing us the ulcer, now smaller, less angry looking, and also much less painful. It took time, but the salve healed that ulcer. Another woman came in with plantar fasciitis and decided to soak her foot nightly in a strong, hot tea made with comfrey root while taking a homeopathic formula containing comfrey as well. She was surprised by the results, as was her doctor.

In the 1970s comfrey was going to save the world. At a certain point, people were eating it at every meal, drinking comfrey tea, and making rope and clothing from the sturdy fiber in the stems. Unfortunately, scientists found hepatotoxic pyrrolizidine alkaloids in comfrey. Many plants can cause big problems if we use too much of them, and comfrey turned out to be damaging livers, particularly in people who had compromised livers for some other reason. There is currently a lot of controversy about the internal use of comfrey. For those just starting out, it is best to be cautious and use minimal amounts.

Having said that, there are a few instances involving internal bleeding of the digestive system or bowels where I might still choose to use comfrey internally. That would be my own decision, and where once I might have used the root, now I would choose only very young leaves. You will find herbalists who put no restrictions on internal use, and you will find herbalists who would never take comfrey internally. I fall somewhere in the middle, but again, only with small, young leaves and for short-term use on an acute condition where the liver is not compromised by another condition.

For instance, many years ago a friend who thought she was dealing with inflammatory bowel disease had a sudden onset of Crohn's disease so severe that she was scheduled for surgery within a month. She asked if we could make a tea that she could use in the meantime to help control the bleeding. After discussing the pros and cons of comfrey, and considering that it was a short-term situation, we made her a tea of comfrey, marshmallow, nettles, and raspberry leaf. It made a huge difference, stopping the bleeding within a few days and enabling her to go into surgery stronger.

In all treatment options there is a risk/benefit decision to make. It is always wise to learn as much as you can about your own situation so that it is easier to weigh those decisions. In our shop and in this book, I do not diagnose or attempt to treat people, but rather suggest what we have learned for our own issues. People who become educated and involved in their own treatment tend to be more optimistic and very often have better outcomes.

Comfrey is also a very good friend to the organic gardener. Rich in nitrogen, potassium, and phosphorus, it beats well-rotted animal manure and commercial fertilizer just about every time. If you're throwing expense into that equation, there is no comparison at all. For fruiting trees, comfrey's silica, calcium, iron, and magnesium, along with other essential nutrients, make it a good choice to use as mulch. In the compost pile, comfrey activates the process and heats up the pile, expediting the decomposition while enriching the compost with its nutrients.

Medicinal Benefits

» Speeds wound healing
» Eases pain
» Staunches internal bleeding
» Heals skin infections
» Treats bruises

COMFREY SALVE

HEALING HERBS

One of the most basic herbal preparations to have in the house is comfrey salve. To make it, you must first infuse an oil with comfrey. There are many different options on how to infuse an oil. Please see page 11 for instructions.

Ingredients

3½ ounces (100 ml) comfrey-infused oil

½ ounce (14 g) beeswax

Up to 40 drops lavender or tea tree essential oil, or a combination of the two (optional)

Directions

In a saucepan over low heat, slowly heat about half the oil with the beeswax until the wax is dissolved. Drizzle in the rest of the oil while stirring constantly. If you'd like to add any essential oils, stir that in while the salve is still liquid.

Pour into a clean, 4-ounce (120 ml) jar. When the salve sets up, put the lid on it and it's ready for use on well-cleaned scratches, bruises, rashes, and sores.

Yield » 4 ounces (120 ml)

COMFREY AND ALOE LOTION

This lotion is terrific for windburn, brush burns, and sunburn. To make the tincture, fill a jar loosely with comfrey leaves and cover with 100 proof alcohol for at least 2 weeks, using a lid on the jar. Please see page 12 for instructions.

Ingredients

1 ounce (28 g) comfrey tincture

3 ounces (84 g) aloe gel (or fresh peeled aloe run through a food processor)

30 drops lavender essential oil

Directions

Blend all the ingredients together very well. Pour into a clean bottle and store in the refrigerator. The chill will be refreshing and soothing on any kind of burn.

Yield » 4 ounces (112 g)

COMFREY ORGANIC FERTILIZER

There are a couple of different methods for this. Both will smell pretty bad, so you'll want to do them outside. Comfrey fertilizer is best used after the first blossoms have set to support the growth of the fruit, seeds, and flowers.

Comfrey Fertilizer Concentrate

This method requires two containers, one larger than the other, with a few holes drilled in the bottom of the smaller container. The drilled container should be able to hold at least a gallon (3.8 L). The second container should be large enough to hold a few gallons of fresh comfrey leaves.

Ingredients

Comfrey leaves

Directions
Stack the comfrey leaves like pieces of paper in the smaller container with the drilled holes. Weight them down with a layer of bricks. Place the container with the comfrey on top of the other, larger container. In a few weeks, the comfrey will decompose, and a black, dreadful-smelling goo will drain into the bottom container.

This is very concentrated, and should be diluted about 15:1 with water.

Comfrey Fertilizer Tea

To make this, use a large container (at least 5 gallons [19 L]).

Ingredients

Comfrey leaves

Directions
Submerge comfrey leaves in water (1 part leaves to 4 or 5 parts water) to rot for about a month. The resulting "tea" is quite concentrated, so dilute it at least 4 to 1 with water.

BOO-BOO SALVE

My friend Susanna Reppert Brill offers these salve instructions. Her daughter loves and rides horses, so Susanna sometimes includes horse manure with the comfrey to make the tea. She loves to tell this story: "I grew up in the herb gardens behind The Rosemary House, quietly absorbing herbal facts and lore as my mother answered endless questions from customers. One year as I was packing to go away to church camp, I packed my swimsuit, T-shirts, shorts, and so on with several large comfrey leaves on top. My mother came in to make sure I had packed undies and my toothbrush, saw the leaves, and asked what they were for. I replied, 'For my boo-boos.' She told me later that she often wondered what those camp counselors thought!"

Ingredients

¼ **cup dried comfrey leaves**

¼ **cup dried yarrow leaves**

¼ **cup dried calendula blossoms**

¼ **cup dried plantain leaves**

2 cups (470 ml) olive oil

1 ounce (28 g) beeswax, grated

10 drops lavender essential oil

10 drops vitamin E oil (optional)

Directions

Combine the herbs in a jar, pour the olive oil over, mix well, and infuse for 2 weeks. You can gently heat the olive oil if you would like to, but it is not necessary.

After 2 weeks, strain the mixture through a piece of cheesecloth or muslin. Press the excess oil out of the herbs.

In a double boiler, add the comfrey oil, beeswax, lavender essential oil, and vitamin E oil and melt together. Once melted, take a small spoonful of the oil and allow it to harden. If it is too soft, add more beeswax. If it is too hard, add more olive oil. If it is perfect, bottle in small jars and label.

Use generously on cuts, scrapes, wounds (not puncture wounds), brush burns, diaper rash, bug bites, poison ivy, and other skin conditions. Salves generally have a shelf life of 3 years or so.

Yield » 12 ounces (355 ml)

Source Susanna Reppert Brill, The Rosemary House, www.TheRosemaryHouse.com

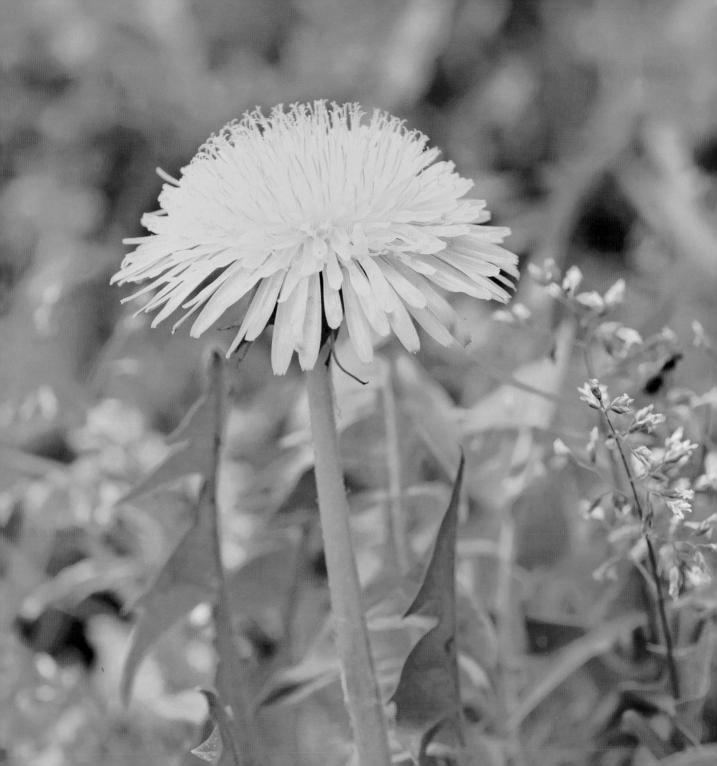

CHAPTER SIXTEEN

Dandelion

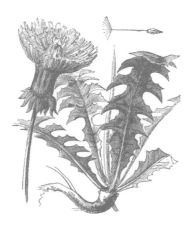

Taraxacum officinale

Asteraceae family

As children, most of us proudly plucked this sunny yellow blossom as an early spring bouquet for our mothers. By the time we got to the house with our treasure, the blooms had closed up, hiding the petals, which were never to open again. When the seed heads develop, the pale white, perfectly round orbs carry our wishes on the wind. Some believe that you must catch a seed in the air to make a wish.

This hardy perennial grows wild in temperate regions. Dandelions grow from rosettes, formed tightly over the root in a crown from which the flower buds are tucked tightly into the center at first, and then burst into view as the leaves grow ever wider. Each seed head has around 200 seeds, with a germination rate of close to 90 percent. Flowers turn to ripe seeds in nine to twelve days. As much as people fight them, dandelions are good for your lawn. Deep, strong, and wide reaching, their roots loosen hard-packed soil, aerate the earth, and help reduce erosion. They pull nutrients up from the soil to fertilize the lawn. More important than ever before, dandelion flowers are a bountiful early source of food for honeybees and butterflies. The roots can grow several feet deep and the plants can live for ten to twelve years. As long as there is sunshine available, the dandelions will persist, so we might as well make friends.

I do nothing to discourage them. During the rainy springtime, there is nothing quite as satisfying as pulling the thick, juicy taproots from the soil, complete and luscious. Before they send up flower stalks, they are excellent to gather. It becomes quite a bit more difficult in dry weather. I harvest them again in the fall, after they've had a summer to gather energy.

Dandelion was such an important vegetable and herb that seeds were brought to the United States by the pilgrims on the Mayflower. The plant is native to Eurasia and has been found in prehistoric deposits in the United States. Many of the herbs that we call weeds today escaped from colonial gardens. The name comes from the appearance of the leaves, lion's tooth, or *dent de lion*. The Latin name (*Taraxacum officinale*) means "official remedy of disorders," and a French nickname, *pissenlit*, which loosely translates to "wet the bed," refers to its diuretic properties.

The fresh spring greens of dandelion acted to clear out the excesses of winter's heavy foods. After months of starches, heavy meats, and roots, the vitamins and minerals are most welcome and the cleansing action fights sluggish blood. The leaves typically become bitter as they grow, but blanching them by blocking them from sunlight renders them a tender delicacy. Blanch them by placing slightly elevated boards above the plants with just enough room to rise from the soil and spread their leaves, but not allowing the sun to reach them. Don't think they need to be blanched, though—the young green leaves are delicious as is. Once the plant has flowered, the leaves become quite bitter, so gather them young. Cooking also decreases the bitterness. We need bitter tastes to stay healthy. The moment we taste bitter, bile is released and our entire digestive systems moves into gear.

Dandelion greens contain great quantities of beta-carotene, potassium, iron, calcium, B vitamins, magnesium, and fiber. The leaves, eaten or brewed into tea, are one of the few potassium-sparing natural diuretics, making it valuable to those fighting edema. It helps cleanse the liver and kidneys and even clears up skin problems in the process.

The roots of dandelion are part two of this blockbuster herb. In spring and fall, our yard and gardens are filled with dandelion. In weeding, the goal is to get the taproot so that the weed does not spread. What luck! We get some great medicine while weeding. To prepare the roots for beverages and storage, clean well, chop or grind coarsely, and roast in a 200°F (93°C) oven until fragrant, darkened, and dry (generally a couple of hours).

All parts of the plant have been used for millennia to treat anemia, scurvy, and skin problems; to promote bile production and digestion; to lower blood pressure, blood sugar, and cholesterol; to relieve inflammation; to ease PMS; and to support the immune system. Dandelion helps maintain regular elimination. The white sap, or latex, exuded from the leaves and stems can be applied to common warts to dissolve them.

Dandelion leaves and roots are available commercially. You can get it in tea form, in tincture, loose/bulk, or in blends used as coffee substitutes. The roasted roots make a very tasty, healthy coffeelike beverage.

The sunny yellow flowers are often overlooked, but they have many uses. Dandelion wine is made with the flowers. They can be made into a beautiful jelly. In omelets, fritters, or salads they add a special something, and the small, tight buds are best when cooked.

Medicinal Benefits

» Promotes urination
» Aids digestion
» Clears skin
» Lowers blood pressure and cholesterol
» Reduces inflammation
» Boosts immunity
» Eases PMS

DANDELION FLOWER-INFUSED OIL

A surprising use of the flowers is in an oil infusion for external use, to relax tight muscles and repair rough skin. I like to use coconut oil for this because it is clear when melted and white when hard. That lets me see the pale yellow left by the petals. There are many ways to infuse oils, but my favorite is in the oven on the lowest setting. Especially when using fresh botanicals in oil, this rapid method with low heat helps keep bacteria at bay so that the oil will remain fresher longer.

Ingredients

1 cup dandelion petals
2 cups (470 ml) melted coconut oil

Directions

On a clear morning, harvest a quart (1 L) or so of whole flowers. Trim out just the yellow parts until you have a heaping cup of bright petals. It isn't critical that they are perfect, but you want as much color as possible. Spread the petals out to wilt for a few hours to evaporate some moisture. Measure 1 cup of the petals.

Combine the petals and the oil in a baking dish with a lot of surface area; a square glass cake pan works well for this. Place in the oven set on the lowest setting, or in a gas oven the pilot light will be sufficient. Several hours (or overnight) later, the oil will be ready.

Strain it carefully and put it into a wide-mouthed jar. The coconut oil will become firm, so in this case a bottle will not work.

Yield » 2 cups (470 ml)

DANDELION VINEGAR

Vinegar is one of the best ways to draw out the minerals in plants. Use the vinegar in cooking or dressings, and all of the benefits are at your fingertips. Choose good-quality vinegar. I always use apple cider vinegar.

Ingredients

1 quart dandelion flowers, leaves, and roots, chopped

1½ quarts (1.4 L) vinegar, or more to cover

Directions

Loosely fill a container with clean chopped leaves, flowers, and roots. I use nearly all leaves and flowers with just a small handful of chopped roots. Cover completely with vinegar. Close with a nonreactive canning lid, and allow to steep for 3 weeks or more. Strain and bottle, and it's ready to use.

Yield » 1 quart

Note

If you notice a bit of white residue, it is the inulin from the root and is harmless.

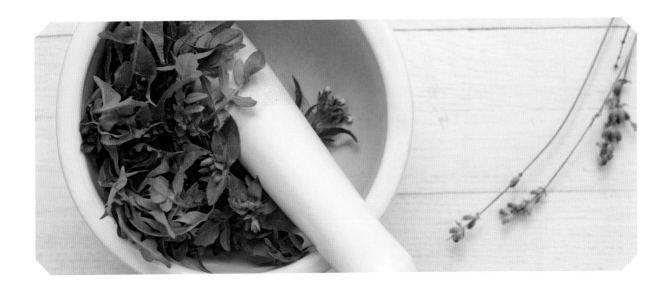

GREEN EGGS

A favorite way to incorporate dandelion greens into a meal is in an egg scramble. In the early spring, this versatile recipe includes lots of wild greens. The tender young leaves and tight buds of dandelion go well with chickweed, and it's often easy to find a tiny wild onion or two. Add a little ham, and you have a literary classic that even a persnickety child might be willing to try.

Ingredients

1 teaspoon unsalted butter

1 cup (70 g) mixed, chopped dandelion greens (may substitute other wild greens or spinach)

3 eggs

1 tablespoon (15 ml) water

Directions

Heat the butter in a skillet and sauté the greens until just slightly wilted and vibrant in color.

Mix together the eggs and water with a fork until uniform, and pour over the greens. Stir together over the heat so that the greens are well mixed into the eggs, and then allow to cook until eggs are set. Turn over once so that both sides are lightly browned.

Yield » 2 servings

Option

There are so many things you can add to this to create a meal, but some of my favorites are grated cheese, chopped onions, garlic, salsa, and ham.

PMS TEA

Keep this blend on hand so that it's ready when you are.

Ingredients

¼ cup dried dandelion leaves

¼ cup dried raspberry leaves

¼ cup dried lemon balm

¼ cup dried spearmint

Directions

Blend the dried herbs together well. Use 1 to 2 teaspoons in a tea ball or muslin bag per cup of tea. Pour the boiling water over the herbs and allow to steep for 5 minutes. Drink as needed.

Yield » Enough for 25 to 30 cups brewed tea

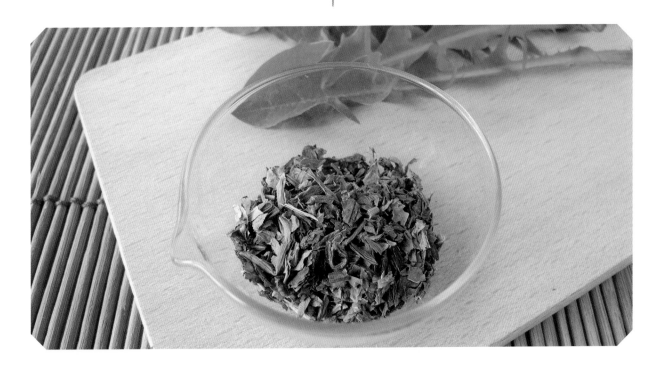

DANDELION FRITTERS

The flowers close quickly after being picked, so this is a great dish if there are children about to keep a supply of the freshly picked blossoms coming into the kitchen. Small children will particularly enjoy gathering for this because you want no stems. They can just pop off the heads and put them in a basket. It works best in small batches.

Ingredients

3 cups dandelion flower heads
1 egg
1 cup (235 ml) milk
1 cup (108 g) seasoned bread crumbs
Cooking oil, for frying

Directions

Rinse the flowers in cold, salted water, and then pat dry.

Combine the egg and milk in a bowl. Dip the flowers, one by one, into the egg mixture, and then dredge in the bread crumbs.

Heat the oil in a skillet over medium heat, add the flowers in batches, and fry until lightly browned. Drain on paper towels, and serve while still hot.

Yield » 3 to 6 servings

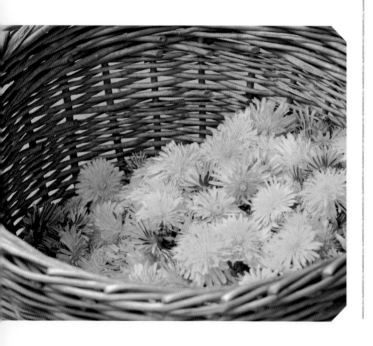

DANDELION ROOT COCOA

Dandelion root cocoa is one of my favorite ways to enjoy dandelion during the winter.

Ingredients

1 quart (1 L) water
¼ cup dandelion root
¼ cup (56 g) roasted raw cacao nibs
1 teaspoon chopped dried reishi mushrooms
3 sticks astragalus root
½ teaspoon ground nutmeg, cinnamon
  or cayenne
1 cup (235 ml) whole milk, coconut milk, or
  almond milk
Raw local honey or stevia, to taste

Directions

Place the water in a saucepan. Add the dandelion, cacao, mushrooms, astragalus, and nutmeg and bring to a boil over medium-high heat. Reduce the heat to a low simmer and cover. Simmer until the liquid is reduced by one-third.

Remove from the heat and strain the herbs from the liquid. Add milk and honey to taste.

Yield » 1 quart (1 L)

Source   Stephany Hoffelt, Naturally Simple Living, www.naturallysimple.org

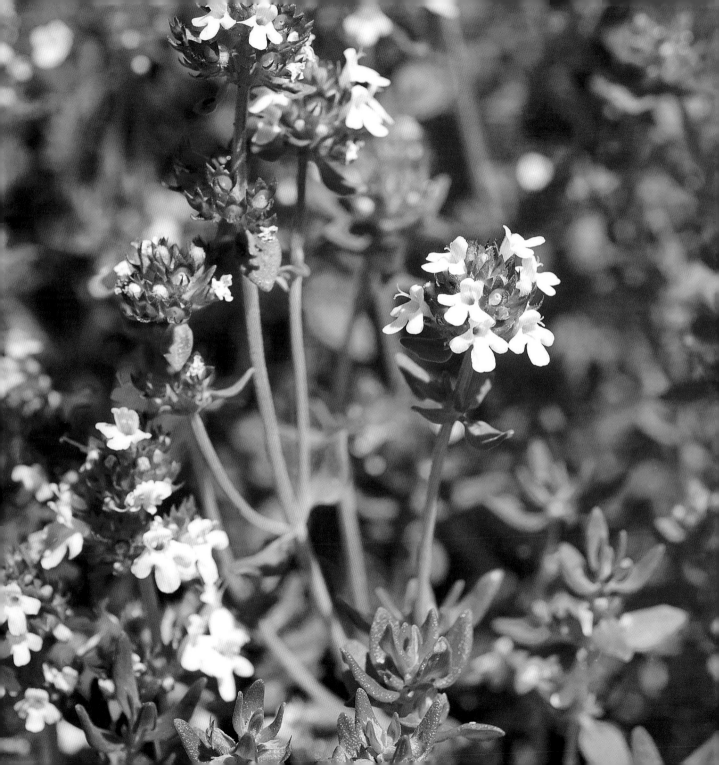

CHAPTER SEVENTEEN

Thyme

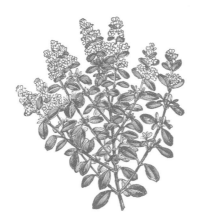

Thymus vulgaris

Labiatae family

Thyme is a seriously overlooked herb. Perhaps due to the diminutive stature, the nearly invisible blossoms, or the fact that it requires almost no care, we tend to forget just how potent this sweet ground cover can be.

In ancient Greece, the word *thymus* meant both "courage" and "to fumigate." Both of these meanings are appropriate to the herb. In medieval times, women gave sprigs of thyme to their knights before they went into battle. Thyme as a form of incense has been used in sickrooms and to purify stale air, and in some cultures it has been used as a perfume. As a strewing herb in the Middle Ages, thyme blended with lavender found its way onto the floors of churches, where it would have helped with musty odors and perhaps kept germs under control.

My friend down the road, Kathy Musser at Cloverleaf Herb Farm, has devoted a large section of her yard to a thyme display garden. When things are in full swing and the thymes are blooming, it is alive with honeybees. You can actually hear them before you round the corner. 'Elfin', 'Creeping', 'Nutmeg', 'Caraway', 'Camphor', 'Wooly', and Mother of Thyme are just a few of the varieties she grows. The blooms are a range of whites, pinks, and pale purples. Depending on the variety, the leaves are anywhere from 1/8 to 1/2 inch (3 to 13 mm) in length, typically about a third as wide as they are long. In other words, they are tiny. The plants form mats of strong, wiry stems that reach across the ground. Rarely do they rise more than a few inches above the soil.

Thyme is one of the most versatile culinary herbs. It can be added to almost any savory dish, and will impart a subtle gourmet quality with little effort. Many of the valuable components are most prevalent in the stems, so chopping up the sprigs and including all aerial parts of the plant is worthwhile. Dried thyme is readily available at the grocery store, but to really enjoy it, grow it or purchase the fresh stems that are available more and more often in the produce section. It is one of the herbs of the fines herbes of French cuisine and is included in the classic bouquet garni or parsley, thyme, and bay leaf.

Thyme is a rich source of nutrition, even in small quantities. It is a treasure trove of vitamins C, B6, K, and A, as well as riboflavin, iron, copper, manganese, calcium, folate, phosphorus, potassium, and zinc. There's even a decent amount of fiber present in thyme. Preparing vinegar with a good quantity of thyme is an excellent way to make those minerals and vitamins available. To do so, simply fill a jar loosely with sprigs of thyme and cover with a good-quality (not distilled) vinegar, allowing it to steep for several weeks in a cool, dark place. Thyme vinegar can be used in many ways. Marinades, dressings, and sauces are delicious, or mix 2 tablespoons (28 ml) of the vinegar with

2 teaspoons (13 g) of blackstrap molasses or honey and ¾ cup (180 ml) of water for a nutrient-packed beverage.

This herb is often vastly overlooked from a home remedy standpoint, making it (along with most culinary herbs) an immensely beneficial and healthful addition to meals. As a carminative herb, it has historically been served to aid digestion, either in the food or as a beverage. The volatile oil components include carvacrol, borneol, and geraniol, but most important is thymol, which can destroy harmful organisms like bacteria, microbes, and viruses and provide antioxidant protection to cellular membranes. Thymol's disinfectant and antiseptic properties can also prevent putrefaction and decay (ancient Egyptians used it in embalming practices).

Using more thyme is a great way to increase the consumption of DHA, an omega-3 fatty acid critical to optimal brain function. Thyme oil is one of several essential oils being studied for its ability to destroy MRSA (Methicillin-resistant Staphylococcus aureus) infections. Scientists have found it to be able to kill this deadly staph infection within two hours. It also shows promise in fighting other deadly bacteria, and it is quite possible that these essential plant oils will be where we turn should antibiotic drugs no longer hold the line. Thyme also includes many flavonoids that work to increase its antioxidant action.

Thyme has a long-standing reputation for treating chest colds and respiratory problems, especially coughs, bronchitis, and congestion. It is an expectorant, helping to loosen excess mucus. It can improve the appetite as well as digestion, and is a remedy for excess gas. A cup of thyme tea can help relieve muscle spasms. It is also diuretic and anti-inflammatory, making it a perfect cup for (among other things) PMS.

Used externally, compresses, soaks, and washes help with a vast array of issues, including acne, scalp problems, athlete's foot and various fungal infections, rashes, bug bites, wounds, and a host of parasites, such as worms, scabies, and lice.

Medicinal Benefits

- » Aids digestion
- » Kills microbes and fungi
- » Kills parasites
- » Inhibits oxidation
- » Disinfects wounds
- » Eases cough
- » Loosens excess mucus
- » Relieves muscle spasms
- » Promotes urination
- » Reduces inflammation

LEMON THYME SHORTBREAD COOKIES

HEALING HERBS

If you've only had thyme in savory dishes, these cookies will open your eyes (and taste buds) to a sweet culinary experience.

Ingredients

½ cup (112 g) unsalted butter, softened

¼ cup (50 g) sugar, plus more for sprinkling

1 tablespoon finely chopped thyme

1 tablespoon (6 g) grated lemon zest

1 tablespoon (15 ml) lemon juice

½ teaspoon crushed cardamom seeds (a mortar and pestle is perfect for this)

1¼ cups (150 g) flour

Directions

Preheat the oven to 350°F (180°C, or gas mark 4).

Using an electric mixer, cream together the butter and sugar until well combined. Add the thyme, lemon zest, lemon juice, and cardamom seed and mix again. Begin adding the flour, mixing in as much as possible with the mixer, but you'll have to work in the rest of it with a spoon or your hands. Work it until it forms a smooth ball.

Divide into 2 portions, and roll out the dough to about ¼-inch (6 mm) thick. Use cutters or a glass to cut out shapes. Sprinkle with sugar and place the cookies on ungreased cookie sheets.

Bake for 12 to 15 minutes, until the edges are lightly browned. Cool on wire racks.

Yield » About 3 dozen cookies

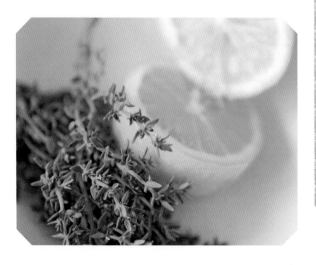

THYME TEA

This can be used as a mouthwash or a gargle, or in larger amounts as a foot soak (add marbles to the basin to rub foot reflexology points). You can add it to bathwater or tent your head over a bowl of steaming tea and inhale as a decongestant.

Ingredients

1 teaspoon dried thyme
1 cup (235 ml) boiling water

Directions

Steep the thyme in the water for 15 minutes. Strain.

Variations

» Add honey to taste and use for colds or upper respiratory problems.
» A lemon slice goes well with thyme and honey for sore throats.
» Add mint and honey for a cough syrup.
» Add a slice of ginger for nausea.

FIRST SIGN OF COLD THYME ELIXIR

Drink this elixir at the first sign of a cold.

Ingredients

½ cup dried thyme
2 slices ginger
1 slice lemon
10 ounces (280 g) honey
5 ounces (140 ml) brandy

Directions

Add the thyme, ginger, and lemon to a 1-pint (470 ml) jar. Add the honey and brandy to cover. Let steep for 6 weeks, then strain and use by the teaspoon or in tea.

Yield » 1 pint (470 ml)

Source
Jackie Johnson, ND, Planhigion Herbal Learning Center, www.planhigion.com, www.thewisconsinherbalist.com

TINCTURE OF THYME

🌿 *This tincture is good at the first sign of a cold. It can also be diluted and used to clean wounds.*

Ingredients

Dried thyme
Brandy or other alcohol

Directions

Fill a 1-pint (470 ml) jar one-third full of dried thyme and add alcohol to fill. Steep for 6 weeks, and then strain and bottle. Take a dropperful, or ½ teaspoon, at a time, up to 3 times a day.

Yield » 1 pint (470 ml)

THYME OIL

🌿 *Oil-infused thyme makes an excellent massage oil for sore joints. Adding lavender and using on the temples eases headaches. See instructions for infusing oil on page 11.*

THYME VINEGAR FOR THE HOME

Directions

Infuse fresh or dried thyme in white vinegar for 2 to 4 weeks. Strain. May be diluted with distilled water. Use to clean floors, counters, windows, and doorknobs.

Source for tincture, oil, vinegar, and oxymel recipes

Jackie Johnson, ND, Planhigion Herbal Learning Center, www.planhigion.com, www.thewisconsinherbalist.com

THYME AND ELDERBERRY OXYMEL

Sip at the first sign of a scratchy throat.

Ingredients

½ cup dried thyme
½ cup dried elderberry
2 or 3 cinnamon chips
2 to 3 ounces (54 to 84 g) honey
Brandy to cover

Directions

Combine the thyme, elderberry, cinnamon, and honey in a 1-pint (470 ml) jar. Mix well. Add brandy to cover. Stir and let sit for 6 weeks. Strain. Use by the teaspoonful. This may be added to other drinks and teas.

Yield » 1 pint (470 ml)

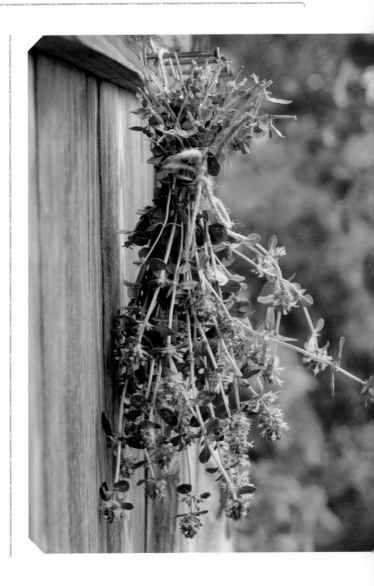

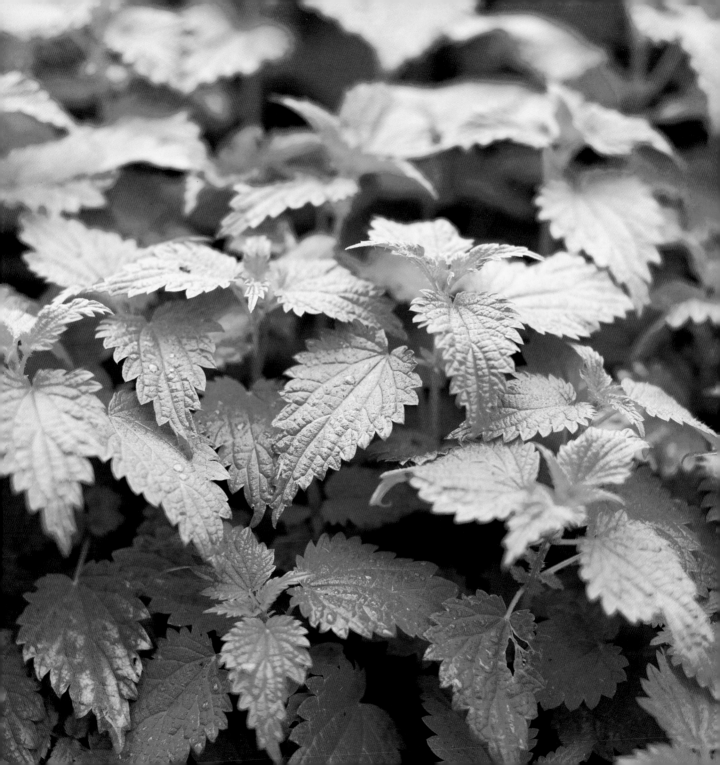

CHAPTER EIGHTEEN

Stinging Nettle

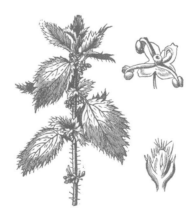

Urtica dioica
Urticaceae family

WHEN MY SISTER and I were children, there was a stream running through a cow pasture where we were allowed to play. All along the stream were patches of stinging nettles, mint, and wild forget-me-nots. Invariably, we would brush against the nettles (which were known to us by the nickname burn hazel), leading us to either jump into the creek to attempt to cool the sting, or just wait it out. The sting doesn't seem to last too long, but it is fierce. After all, its family name, Urticaceae, is derived from the Latin *uro*, to burn. Duration depends on the individual and the plant. We learned very young to recognize this perennial, which can sometimes grow to a height of 7 feet (2 m). Its paired leaves are heart shaped and coarsely veined and sharply toothed, and there is something in the appearance that looks a little mean. Nettle likes damp places and moist ground, and its presence is frequently an indicator of rich soil. The stems and undersides of all the leaves are covered with hollow stinging hairs called trichomes that inject chemicals that can produce welts, redness, and the stinging sensation.

Never in a million years did that child feeling the sting of nettle think that someday it would become a favorite vegetable as well as a valued medicinal herb in our family! There are a few wild vegetables that I love, and stinging nettle is at the top of that list. The flavor somehow conveys well-being when steamed and buttered.

Flavor aside, stinging nettle really is good for you! It contains tannic acid, lecithin, chlorophyll, iron, silica, potassium, phosphorus, sulfur, sodium, and vitamins A and C. The dried leaves contain up to 40 percent protein, so adding the powdered, dried leaves to smoothies, soups, stews, and a thousand other dishes can boost their nutritional content.

Nettle supports chest and upper respiratory complaints and is often a first line of defense against seasonal allergies. Taken with a local honey, nettle can shush away mild to moderate symptoms. It is best to begin using nettle before allergy season gets underway.

Nettle is used in cases of internal and external bleeding and also helps fight anemia and the fatigue that accompanies it due to its readably available iron content and the vitamin C that helps with absorption. The herb is sometimes recommended to help nursing mothers increase milk production. In pregnancy, the mineral-packed herb is good for mother and the developing baby. In fact, nettle is a good, lifelong woman's herb, helping to regulate how the liver processes and eliminates estrogen, smoothing out PMS symptoms, helping to regulate heavy menses, and being an all-around support in menopause. Regular use of nettle may help the body retain more estrogen. Estrogen loss affects memory, bone health, heart health, and skin tone and elasticity, so drink up, ladies!

The sting has been used externally on joints affected with osteoarthritis to relieve pain (a process called urtification), and internal use of nettle in combination with NSAIDs is effective enough that often the use of NSAIDs can be substantially lowered. Those with inflammatory diseases such as arthritis, gout, and rheumatism and soft-tissue conditions such as fibromyalgia and tendonitis find pain relief from daily use. Autoimmune disorders that include joint pain also respond favorably to nettle use. Nettle contains a healthy quantity of the trace mineral boron, which is important in helping bones retain calcium. It is surprisingly healing for the digestive tract as well. Nettle is also effective as a mouthwash against plaque, gingivitis, and mouth sores; helps with sore throats; strengthens mucous membranes; and can assist with acid reflux, celiac disease, gas, colitis, nausea, and swollen hemorrhoids. This amazing weed supports the endocrine system as well.

Nettle is a wonderful spring tonic that helps in the elimination of the metabolic wastes that build up during a winter of being indoors, gently stimulating the lymph system and encouraging the kidneys to move things along efficiently. The seeds are considered energizing, provide adrenal support, and may help with weight loss. The root is used for prostate health and to help

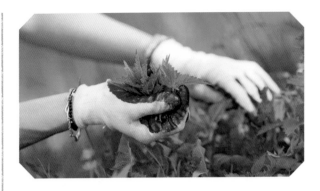

with the urination issues found in men with enlarged prostates. It is diuretic and astringent, and can be useful in joint issues by promoting the release of uric acid from joints. The root is also considered a pelvic decongestant and can be useful for problems with menstruation.

Medicinal Benefits

» Promotes urination
» Constricts tissue
» Alleviates pain
» Stops bleeding
» Alleviates joint pain
» Reduces allergy
» Reduces congestion
» Helps expel excess mucus
» Calms muscle spasm
» Aids digestion

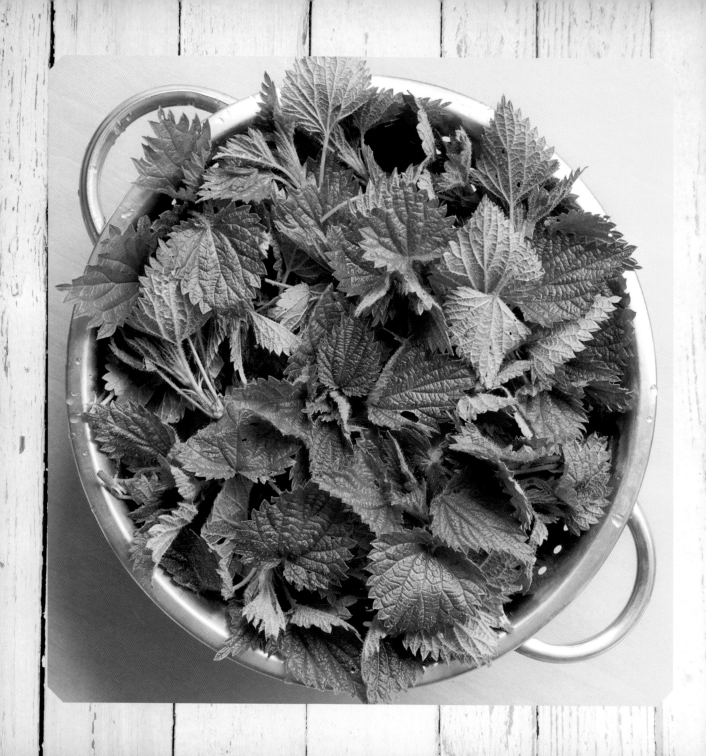

STEAMED NETTLE

By far, my favorite spring dish is a bowl of deep green nettle with a pat of butter and a sprinkle of good sea salt. It is the easiest thing in the world (if you wear protective gloves) and you can almost feel your body welcoming spring while you eat it. Heating the nettle takes the sting away. Drying does too, but I've occasionally been stung by dried nettle, but not with cooked.

Ingredients

½ cup (120 ml) water
1 quart young nettle leaves
Butter and salt to taste

Directions

In a saucepan, bring the water to a boil. Add the nettle leaves, cover, return to a boil quickly, and then reduce the heat to steam the leaves for 3 to 5 minutes. Strain, add butter and salt, and eat.

Yield » 2 servings

NETTLE AND LEEK SOUP

This traditional springtime soup uses some of the first greens of the year.

Ingredients

4 tablespoons (56 g) unsalted butter

1 cup (100 g) chopped leeks

1 quart (1 L) chicken or vegetable broth

4 medium potatoes, sliced (skin on)

1 quart tender young nettle leaves, chopped

Salt and pepper to taste

Sour cream, for garnish

Directions

Melt the butter in large saucepan and add the leeks. Sauté until just tender, 5 or 6 minutes. Add the broth and potatoes and heat to a low boil. When the potatoes are nearly done, add the nettle. Simmer for another 15 minutes. Use a stick blender to purée the soup. I like to leave it a little chunky. A food processor or blender will work too, but I love the convenience of finishing it right in the pan. Add salt and pepper. Serve with a dollop of sour cream in the center of each bowl.

Yield » 4 to 6 servings

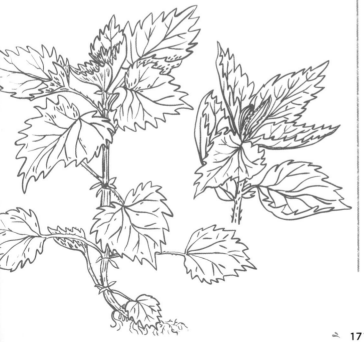

NETTLE HOT OIL HAIR TREATMENT

🌿 *Nettle helps strengthen hair, adds shine, and stimulates hair growth.*

Ingredients

1 cup fresh, wilted, chopped nettle
  (or ½ cup dried)
2 cups (470 ml) jojoba oil
½ teaspoon lavender essential oil
¼ teaspoon rosemary essential oil

Directions

Place the nettles in a mason jar and cover with jojoba oil. Cover the jar with a square of cheesecloth, held in place by the metal ring, so the moisture in the herbs can escape. Place the jar in a sunny, south-facing window and stir well every day for 3 weeks.

To strain, pour the oil through an old T-shirt into a clean jar. When it stops dripping, gather in the corners and twist and squeeze out every last drop. Add the essential oils. Place a lid and screw band on the jar for long-term storage.

To use, massage ½ to 2 teaspoons into the hair, depending on the length, and then brush it well to distribute it. Wrap the hair for about an hour, then shampoo as usual.

Yield » 2 cups (470 ml)

Source   Marci Tsohonis

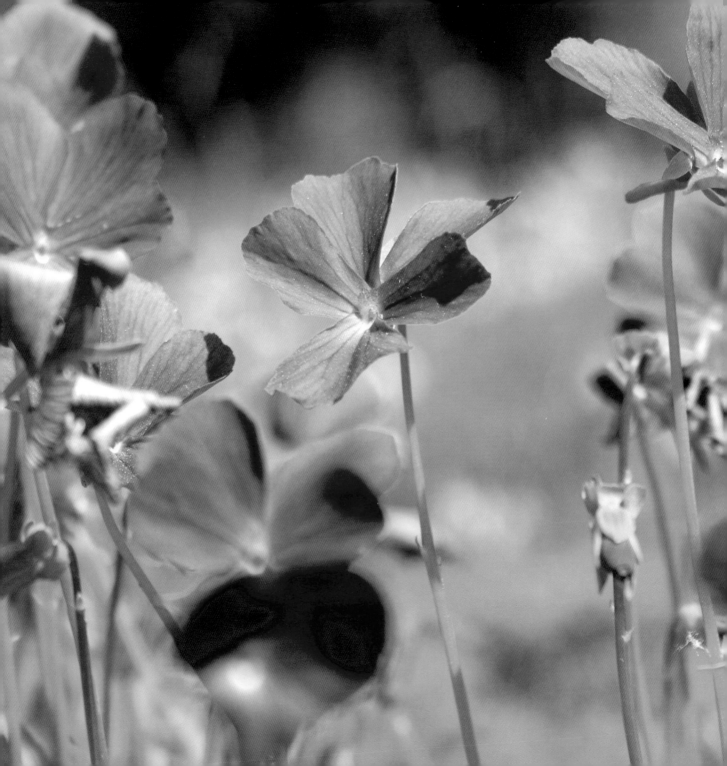

CHAPTER NINETEEN

Sweet Violet

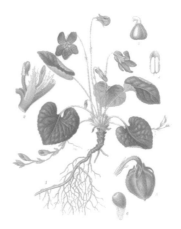

Viola odorata
Violaceae family

Viola odorata is the most common garden violet, growing wild between blades of grass. The flowers have a sweet, powdery scent and are typically either dark violet or white, the emerald heart-shaped leaves and flowers are all in a rosette, and the leaf stalks have hairs that point downward. The flowers rise quickly above the leaves, only to be overtaken by them as their bloom fades. The flowers appear as early as February and last until the end of April. In early fall, you'll find the seedpods opening very close to the earth, like tiny three-pointed stars. There is often a very small bloom in autumn too, made all the sweeter by the impending winter.

Violets hold a very warm spot in my heart. I always looked forward to May Day when I was little, and loved to leave little paper cones full of violets and other flowers on the doorknobs of neighbors (most likely to be found days later). Picking thick bundles of the little flowers is one of the few ways to ever actually smell the scent of their perfume. Another is to pick baskets full for syrup or jelly, put most of your face into the basket and inhale deeply—just one long inhalation. After that, it will be gone. In a very odd trick of nature, sweet violets contain a ketone compound called ionone that temporarily desensitizes the receptors in the nose. You get one sniff. After that, ionone has made it impossible to smell it again for a brief time.

Up until the 1940s violet essential oil was made through an exhaustive and low-yielding method of enfleurage and solvent extraction. Then, synthetic approximations became much more profitable and therefore more commonplace. Violet leaf essential oil is available today; however, it's quite expensive. Every spring or summer, I attempt to distill it myself, but so far it hasn't worked out. I obtain a great hydrosol, but as yet no essential oil.

Violets have a rich history. They were Napoleon's signature flower, and he covered Josephine's grave with them. In ancient Greece violets were the official symbol of Athens, and wines were scented with them. In *Footnotes to the Violet*, John Reismiller writes, "The Greek dramatist, Aristophanes, referred to Athens in one of his plays as the violet-crowned city because the name of the king who was crowned there (Ion) and the flower (ion = violet) were the same. The English historian Macaulay used the same epithet for that ancient city when he wrote of it and it has been emblematic of it ever since." Violet is still the emblem of Toulouse, France. A golden violet is presented today at the Académie Française as an award.

Violet blossoms and leaves are higher in vitamin C than any domestic green vegetable. They also contain vitamin A. Both of those vitamins are very important to immune function and wound healing. I don't see a lot of references to eating these as vegetables in the long-ago history when we lived on the contents of our root cellars and whatever we preserved (as we often see with dandelion), but we should have. There are lots of vital minerals, especially calcium and magnesium, available in the leaves, too. The leaves and flowers contain rutin, a bioflavonoid that is helpful in the treatment of venous insufficiency and lowered blood flow to various parts of the body. Specifically, hemorrhoids and varicose veins may respond to violet.

The leaves especially contain saponins and mucilage. Last year I attempted to distill the tender early green leaves. The steam passing through those delicate leaves changed it into a mass of bubbling goo within half an hour. Removing it from the flask, it was silky, slippery, and mucilaginous. Who says we don't learn anything from our mistakes? The saponins are helpful in dissolving all kinds of lumps and cysts, most traditionally used for the breasts. The mucilage improves the health and moisture of mucous membranes, which helps maintain bowel regularity, supports lung function, and soothes the gastrointestinal and urinary tracts. These qualities also make violet a good, gentle option for dry skin, acne, cradle cap, and eczema. Externally for the skin, it can be used as an infused oil (for dry, scaly skin) or a poultice for conditions such as acne.

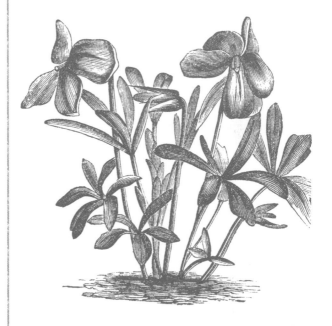

Medicinal Benefits

» Treats skin issues
» Supports gastrointestinal health
» Boosts immune function
» Heals wounds
» Improves blood flow

CANDIED VIOLETS

Although this is painstaking work, the visual delight when candied violets make an appearance on a dish is worth it. There is almost nothing prettier than a cupcake swathed in white frosting with a few candied violets scattered across the top.

Ingredients

Dried violet blossoms, fully open, about 1 inch (2.5 cm) of stem attached
Egg white, beaten, at room temperature
Sugar

Directions

With a small paintbrush, paint each blossom completely with the egg white. Immediately cover with sugar. Place on parchment paper that has been laid over racks in a warm, dry place. Gently snip away the stem. Let dry for 24 hours.

Once dried, store in a clean, dry, airtight container with layers separated by waxed paper or parchment.

Yield » As desired

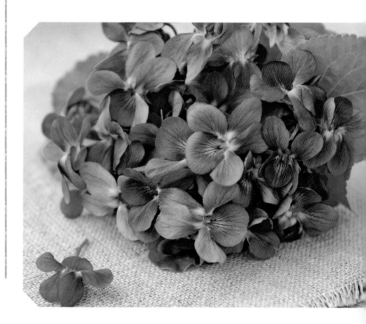

VIOLET SYRUP

I was introduced to this when my daughter, Molly, was in nursery school, and one of the other mothers made it. The color of her syrup was the palest of lavenders, as she'd set her violets in water to bathe under the full moon. It was really lovely, but I usually am in more of a hurry. One of the attractions of violet syrup has to do with the brief window of time that we get to enjoy them and the striking color. Molly and I used to wander down into the orchard and while away entire afternoons popping the blossoms into a wide bowl. I've since learned to use something with more depth and less width—one good gust and the whole afternoon's worth of violets is in the wind.

Ingredients

1 quart lightly packed violet blossoms, without stems

1 dried rose geranium leaf or 1 drop rose geranium essential oil (optional)

3 cups (705 ml) boiling water

Juice of 1 lemon

4 cups (800 g) sugar

Directions

Place the violets in a large heat-resistant jar. If you have a rose geranium leaf, add that. Pour the boiling water over the flowers. Let steep for 1 hour. Strain. Note that the color is likely greenish blue. Wait for it . . . add the lemon juice. Magic! It's purple.

Heat the liquid in a saucepan, add the sugar, stir to combine, and bring to a boil. Boil for 3 minutes, stirring to dissolve the sugar. Cool enough to pour into clean jars. Cover and refrigerate. The sugar is probably enough to preserve it, but use the fridge to be sure. Use this syrup to sweeten teas, brighten up some vanilla ice cream, or splash on sorbet. It's great on crepes and drizzled over strawberries, too.

Yield » 1 quart (1 L)

VIOLET LEAF SALVE

Because violet is such a gentle healer, I like to double or triple infuse the oil used in a salve. In order to do that, I infuse the oil, strain it, add fresh plant material, infuse, strain, repeat. This way, I wind up with a more concentrated salve. Violet leaves are available from spring until early fall, so it's easy to do this. I may have mentioned that I'm not the patient type, so I use my oven on the lowest "warm" setting, allowing me to accomplish a triple-infused oil in a day if I start first thing.

For this one, I like to use coconut oil. Because we're using a little heat, it will be liquid, and since the coconut oil is white, the salve will be a nice green. I like the power of a deep green salve.

Ingredients

½ **cup (120 ml) violet-infused oil**
½ **ounce (14 g) beeswax**

Directions

Make the violet-infused oil (see page 11), then strain carefully, removing any grit, for the last time.

Heat the beeswax very slowly with about ¼ cup (60 ml) of the infused oil until it is liquid. Slowly add the rest of the oil so that the wax doesn't seize. Pour into small, clean wide-mouthed jars. This is a good salve for hands that have been working outside in rough weather or working without gloves in drying clay soils. It's great for older faces and skin, and perfect for sore legs and venous issues.

NETTLE AND WILD VIOLET BODY CREAM

Blue violet has an affinity to the lymphatic system and is classified as an alliterative, or "blood purifier"; it is known to promote the body's own cleansing action. It is a great herb for swollen glands and helping the body eliminate bacteria and other toxins, which is why violets are traditionally known for their use in body and breast care, and also for chapped and dry spots. Here's one of my favorite lusciously clean-smelling creams perfect for thirsty skin. It's light and dreamy and filled with the essence of spring.

Ingredients

1 cup fresh blue violet flowers

3 ounces (90 ml) nettle and violet leaf–infused sunflower oil

½ ounce (15 ml) castor oil

1½ ounces (42 g) shea butter

½ ounce (14 g) grated beeswax

2 vitamin E capsules

5 to 8 drops ylang ylang, jasmine, neroli, or essential oil of choice

Directions

Place the fresh violet flowers into a small heat-proof mason jar and pour hot water over them. Cover and let steep.

Place the nettle and violet leaf–infused oil into a heatproof measuring cup. Add the castor oil, shea butter, and beeswax. Set the cup into a pan filled with several inches of water and heat on medium-low until everything melts together. Remove from the pan, let cool to body temperature, and then add the vitamin E.

Strain the violet flower tea and measure out 5 to 6 ounces (150 to 180 ml) of liquid. Using a hand mixer (or blender) on low, slowly drizzle the violet flower tea into the oil mixture. As the oils start to thicken, increase the speed to high. Beat on high until your mixture is thick and creamy, and then stir in your desired essential oils. Spoon the cream into a clean sterilized jar and enjoy generously!

Yield » 12 ounces (355 ml)

Source
Jessica Morgan, www.MorganBotanicals.com

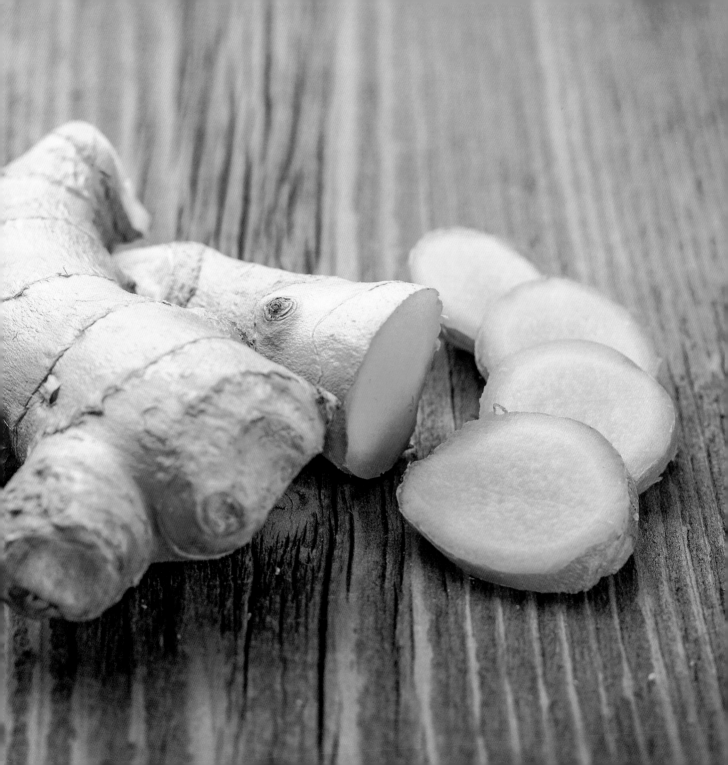

CHAPTER TWENTY

Ginger

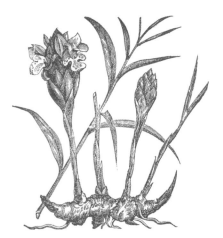

Zingiber officinale
Zingiberaceae family

A<small>T THE MOMENT</small>, there are at least five different concoctions of ginger in my kitchen, and that doesn't count the crystallized ginger that is always on hand, or the granulated spicy hot Chinese honey ginger instant brew that is one of our go-to warm-ups on chilly winter nights.

Ginger is native to Southeast Asia, and it has been renowned for millennia in many areas of the world. Ginger is mentioned in ancient Chinese, Indian, and Middle Eastern writing, and is revered for its aromatic, culinary, and medicinal properties. Ancient Romans imported ginger from China nearly 2,000 years ago. In the 1500s, ginger's use spread, in spite of the great expense of importing it from Asia. Spanish explorers took ginger to the West Indies, Mexico, and South America, and in the sixteenth century exports back to Europe commenced to satisfy the great demand. Jamaica, India, Fiji, Indonesia, and Australia grow most of what we use today. Even though almost every other plant in this book is generally thought of as a weed and can likely be found wild in most temperate regions, ginger is included because it can easily be grown right in the kitchen. It takes a year or two to grow a steady source, but it's worth it. Here's how:

1. First you need some really good soil. Ginger will grow in rich soil that retains moisture, but there must also be good drainage. You won't want the soil to dry out between waterings, but it should be moist, not soggy.

2. Choose fresh plump "hands" from the grocer, and soak overnight. They can be cut into pieces or planted whole. A 12-inch (30.5 cm) diameter pot will handle about three good-size hands.

3. Plant them 3 inches (7.5 cm) deep with the buds facing up.

4. Place the pot where there is good sunlight, but not in direct light; it doesn't have to hog all your good windowsill space.

5. Once established, you can just dig up what you need when you want it. It's best to leave it alone for a year to get it well established, though.

To freeze leftover ginger, grate the ginger thoroughly. Add a teaspoon or two of water or lemon juice, just to increase moisture. Press firmly into ice cube trays, and freeze. When frozen, pop them out and place into a freezer bag, squeezing out the excess air. Now you have ginger ready when you need it.

There are many gingers in the Zingiberaceae family. The three most common are *Zingiber officinale*, which is the traditional ginger; *Curcuma longa*, known as turmeric;

and *Alpinia galanga*, called galangal. Of these three, ginger and turmeric have been found in recent years to have almost unlimited benefits for human health, offering cures for everything from an upset stomach to quite possibly curing or preventing cancer. I expect that very soon we'll be learning more about benefits from galangal. These roots are spectacular, incredibly health-giving, and deliciously easy to add to the diet every single day. Other significant up-and-coming gingers are cardamom (*Elettaria carda-momum*) and zedoary (*Curcurma zedoaria*).

Since discovering ginger's ability to clear nausea almost instantly, I rarely suffer from it as long as I have ginger at hand. I offered a cousin taking a cruise a baggie of ginger root capsules with instructions to use them if she got seasick. Some days into the trip, the ship hit rough seas. She later told me that she was one of very few out and about on the decks.

When added to other herbs—in teas, tinctures, or syrups, for instance—ginger activates them. Ginger is a stimulant, and it promotes circulation, helping to get things moving. It is a highly effective anti-inflammatory, and because inflammation is behind so much lethal diseases, especially in our blood vessels and major organs, ginger can be very useful. Antibiotic and antibacterial, it fights staph infections and might be useful (preemptively) against effects of gamma radiation. It is also antifungal.

Ginger offers pain relief in much the same way cayenne does, and can be used externally in balms, salves, and liniments on sore joints and muscles. Used internally for pain, ginger extract has been shown to be as effective as ibuprofen for menstrual pain and as good as or better than some of the pharmaceutical drugs used for gout, osteoarthritis in the knees, and rheumatoid arthritis, without the toxic side effects. It supports heart health as well. And, it is delicious! Few baked sweets go into our oven without some finely minced crystallized ginger blended into the batter first. It brightens up almost everything.

There are some drug interactions to be aware of when using ginger regularly or in large quantity, so discuss it with your physician if you are using heart medications, NSAIDS, medication for diabetes, or a blood-thinning medication.

Medicinal Benefits

- » Treats nausea
- » Promotes circulation
- » Reduces inflammation
- » Kills bacteria, fungi, and other pathogens
- » Relieves pain (internal and external)

SPICY GINGER ELIXIR

I started making this when there was leftover ginger. In the beginning, it was just a ginger tincture (see page 12 for tincture instructions), but it gradually became this delicious blend that can be taken alone by the dropperful, or added to hot water or herbal tea to jazz it up with healthful properties. It has never had an exact recipe, but this is a good starting point.

Ingredients

½ cup (50 g) chopped ginger
1 lemon, thinly sliced
1 (4-inch, or 10 cm) cinnamon stick
2 star anise
2 cardamom pods
½ cup (160 g) raw local honey
1 cup (235 ml) 100 proof vodka or brandy

Directions

Place the ginger, lemon slices, cinnamon, star anise, cardamom and honey into a pint jar, stir to combine, and add the vodka to cover (it may take a bit more or less than 1 cup [235 ml]). Allow to steep for about a month. Strain into a clean jar and enjoy.

Yield » 1 cup (235 ml)

HEALTHY MORNING MUFFINS

These bran muffins contain no sugar, but with the applesauce and banana you won't notice. There's lots of nourishing goodness here to start the day on an even note. They freeze well, too.

Ingredients

1 cup (120 g) wheat bran

1 cup (120 g) oat bran

1 cup (120 g) whole wheat flour

2 teaspoons baking powder

1 teaspoon baking soda

2 tablespoons (12 g) minced fresh ginger

½ teaspoon cinnamon

½ teaspoon nutmeg

1 cup (245 g) applesauce

1 mashed ripe banana

½ cup (120 ml) skim milk

2 egg whites, lightly beaten

2 tablespoons (30 ml) olive oil

Directions

Preheat the oven to 400°F (200°C, or gas mark 6). Line a 12-cup muffin tin with paper liners.

In a large bowl, combine the wheat and oat brans, whole wheat flour, baking powder, baking soda, ginger, cinnamon, and nutmeg. In another bowl, combine the applesauce, banana, milk, egg whites, and oil. Pour the wet ingredients into the dry ingredients and mix until just combined. Divide evenly among the prepared muffin cups.

Bake for 14 to 16 minutes, or until a toothpick inserted into the center comes out sticky but not wet. Cool on a wire rack.

Yield » 12 muffins

BANANA GINGER BREAD

The ginger adds sparkle to the flavors in this cakelike bread, making it a favorite at our house.

Ingredients

2 cups (240 g) all-purpose flour
¾ teaspoon baking soda
½ teaspoon salt
½ cup (100 g) sugar
¼ cup (56 g) unsalted butter, softened
2 large eggs
1½ cups (338 g) mashed ripe banana (about 3 bananas)
¼ cup (80 g) plain yogurt
2 tablespoons minced crystallized ginger
1 teaspoon vanilla extract

Directions

Preheat the oven to 350°F (180°C, or gas mark 4). Grease an 8½ x 4½-inch (21.5 x 11.5 cm) loaf pan.

Combine the flour, baking soda, and salt in a bowl and stir with a whisk. With a mixer, cream the sugar and butter together in a large bowl. Add the eggs, 1 at a time, beating well after each addition. Add the banana, yogurt, ginger, and vanilla. Blend well.

Add the flour mixture slowly and beat at low speed just until moist. Spoon the batter into the prepared pan. Bake for 1 hour, or until a wooden toothpick inserted into the center comes out clean.

Cool in the pan on a wire rack for 10 minutes. Remove from the pan and cool completely on the wire rack.

Yield » 1 loaf

Note

If using fresh minced ginger root, increase the sugar by ¼ cup (50 g).

GINGER MINT LINIMENT

🌿 *My favorite use for this liniment is on tired feet and calves after a long day of standing.*

Ingredients

¼ cup (25 g) grated fresh ginger
1¼ cups (295 ml) olive oil
5 to 10 drops peppermint essential oil

Directions

Heat the ginger and the olive oil together over the lowest heat setting for up to an hour. Remove from the heat and allow to rest overnight. Strain the cooled oil through a coffee filter to remove all solids. Add the essential oil. Pour into bottles. Massage into sore areas gently to relieve pain.

Yield » 1 cup (235 ml)

GINGER BATH

🌿 *This energizing soak will help with tired, sore muscles.*

Ingredients

1 cup (100 g) grated or sliced ginger

Directions

Place the ginger in a muslin bag and tie securely. Place the muslin bag in a tub of hot water and steep for 10 minutes. Or, attach the bag to the faucet and allow hot water to run through it. Soak in the hot bath for 20 to 30 minutes.

Yield » 1 application

Source
Heddy Johannesen, www.heddyjohannesen.wordpress.com

Metric Conversions

These weights and measures will vary according to the form of the herb used, the moisture content, and how it has been processed. Commercially cut and sifted dry herb that is stored in high humidity will weigh a good deal more than that which has been home-dried and hand-crushed by someone living in an arid climate. Fresh herbs will also vary in weight depending on when they were harvested (just in from the garden, or sent to market the day before yesterday), growing conditions, and whether they are chopped finely or coarsely.

Fortunately, folk herbalism is very forgiving and most of the measurements are not critical, but merely provide a guideline.

4 ounces volume converted to grams

Herb	Dry	Fresh
ashwagandha	0.65 ounce	1.85 ounce
basil	4	8
calendula	3	7
California poppy	6	13
catnip	5	8
chamomile	4	7
chickweed	2	5
chives	4	20
comfrey	7	16
crystallized ginger	7	n/a
dandelion leaf	2	4

Herb	Dry	Fresh
dandelion petals	3	8
dandelion root	27	70
dried nettle	3	n/a
dried thyme	2 to 3	5
elderberry	30	74
elderflowers	2	2
frankincense	54	n/a
gotu kola	12	1
garlic scapes	n/a	22
hops	2	5
lavender buds	6	9
lemon balm	5	7
oat straw/milky oats	13	25
parsley	16	30
motherwort	3	7
passionflower	10	21
peppermint	5	7
plantain	3	11
raspberry leaves	2	8
red clover blossoms	4	6
rose petals	4	8
saw palmetto	44	n/a?
sage	4	10
skullcap	6	8
spearmint	5	7
turmeric	54 powder	104
valerian root	28	70
violet flowers	5	8
violet leaves	4	9
wilted nettle	n/a	8 wilted
yarrow	3	7

Index

Acknowledgments

MANY THANKS to Bob Schwartz for using all the farm equipment to turn our visions into reality, and keeping a clear path into the woods. You're always there, ready to help.

Thanks to Elwin Warner for reminding me why I do what I do whenever the urge to throw in the towel strikes. For thirteen years of encouragement and loving shoves, thank you.

To Maryanne Schwartz, the sister with whom I apparently share a brain. You come along on all the adventures, keep me from leaping out of moving cars at the sight of unusual wildflowers, and make me think that I can accomplish things that seem impossible.

Thank you Molly Sams, for stepping into my shoes this year, taking the herb courses, learning the business, and taking so much weight off my shoulders. Especially, thank you for growing up around the scattered pages, the long hours of being on your own because of my work, and your constant willingness to pitch in. You'll never know how proud I am to be your mom.

To the many herbalists and herb enthusiasts who have been a part of my education and passion for herbs over the years. There are too many to mention, but I'd especially like to thank Susanna Reppert Brill for nearly thirty years of sage advice and encouragement. To all of the herbalists who contributed recipes and remedies to these chapters—thank you, and thank you for your friendship.

Finally, to Esther Snyder. Thanks, Mom, for teaching us about . . . well, everything.

About the Author

TINA SAMS is the editor of *The Essential Herbal* magazine. After many years of running wholesale and retail herb businesses, she decided to pull together some of those resources and friends made during those careers into an herb magazine, with the goal of helping aspiring herbalists connect and share information together. Currently in its thirteenth year of publication, the magazine continues to educate and inspire. Wildcrafting herbs and wild edibles are of vast interest to Tina, as well as soapmaking, medicinal and culinary uses of herbs, distilling essential oils and hydrosols, and various herb crafts. Based in Lancaster County, Pennsylvania, Tina Sams lives and works with her daughter Molly on her sister's family tree farm, and can be reached through her website at www.essentialherbal.com.

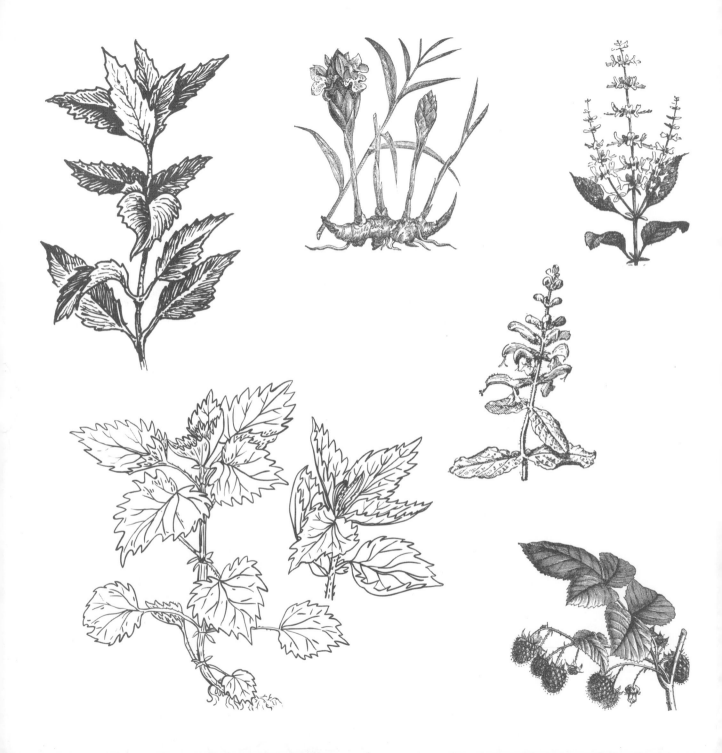